ROOPA FAROOKI is a writer and a junior doctor in the NHS. She is the author of eight books, which have been translated into over a dozen languages, and is the recipient of the John C. Laurence Prize from the Authors' Foundation, for writing that improves understanding between cultures, and an Arts Council Award. She is also a lecturer on the Oxford University Masters in Creative Writing and is Ambassador for Relate (relate.org.uk), the counselling charity. In 2020 she was awarded the Junior Doctor Leadership Prize for her work during the Covid pandemic from her NHS Trust, and the Merit Certificate in the category of clinical excellence from her Deanery. She was shortlisted for Junior Doctor of the Year 2021–2022. Born in Lahore, Pakistan, she lives and works in south-east England.

@RoopaFarooki

@Relate_charity

Everything is True

A Junior Doctor's Story of Life, Death and Grief in a Time of Pandemic

Dr Roopa Farooki

BLOOMSBURY PUBLISHING

LONDON · OXFORD · NEW YORK · NEW DELHI · SYDNEY

BLOOMSBURY PUBLISHING
Bloomsbury Publishing Plc
50 Bedford Square, London, WC1B 3DP, UK
29 Earlsfort Terrace, Dublin 2, Ireland

BLOOMSBURY, BLOOMSBURY PUBLISHING and the Diana logo are
trademarks of Bloomsbury Publishing Plc

First published in Great Britain 2022
This edition published 2023

A catalogue record for this book is available from the British Library

ISBN: PB: 978-1-5266-3341-5; EBOOK: 978-1-5266-3336-1;
EPDF: 978-1-5266-3340-8

2 4 6 8 10 9 7 5 3 1

Typeset by Newgen KnowledgeWorks Pvt. Ltd., Chennai, India
Printed and bound in Great Britain by CPI Group (UK) Ltd, Croydon CR0 4YY

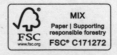

To find out more about our authors and books visit www.bloomsbury.com
and sign up for our newsletters

For my sister, Kiron

And for all those who have lost someone they love

'After you have read this story of great misfortune, you will blame the author for your own insensitivity, accusing of wild exaggeration and flights of fancy. But rest assured: this tragedy is not a fiction. Everything is true.'

Honoré de Balzac, *Le Père Goriot*

Quarantine: originally defined as a period of forty (*quarante* in French, *quaranta* in Italian) days of isolation to prevent the spread of contagious disease.

PROLOGUE: *Six Months Before Lockdown...*

... your sister tells you that she's dying, at her kitchen table, with the sunshine streaming in from her expensive wall of French windows, and there's not much you can say to that.

A little bit of you wishes that you hadn't turned up so dutifully, that you'd made any feeble family-avoiding excuse, because she wouldn't have told you in a text message or on the phone. Not again, anyway. She'd done that before, a couple of times, actually, about matters of life and death, and it hadn't gone well. Sadly, spiralling dark news comes out as weirdly comic when you're separated by a screen. Holding a handset. She'd called you one morning, sixteen years earlier, when you both worked in Berkeley Square in big offices that were minutes from each other, and came straight out with this:

They said Dad's dead. A glittering thread of disbelieving humour in her voice.

They said what? Matching disbelief in yours, admiration, even, that your dad had managed to fake his death and saddle some poor corpse with his debts. You both didn't think that he would do anything so mundane as to die.

Dad's dead. Sure. You'd both laughed, and you had never since admitted that inappropriate laugh to each other. You'd kept a guilty, conspiratorial silence. No need to think about that again, you'd written about it before. And it's not about that, anymore.

I've got breast cancer, she'd messaged you, ten years ago. They're taking off my boob.

You'd just had twins. She'd known about the cancer weeks before she told you, but it was towards the end of your pregnancy, so she waited for you to deliver the babies before she delivered her news. Drop babies, drop the headline. Breaking water, breaking news. Like that was logical. Like it was better. For you or for her.

You'd read her message between three-hour feeds, the babies squalling with open mouths like beaked birds in a nest.

When she didn't answer your frantic calls and you got emotional on Messenger, she texted tersely back.

You need to chill. It's not about you.

That was ten years ago. The first diagnosis. That was then, and this is now.

So you knew already. About her dying of breast cancer. Of course you did. And we're all dying, right? Just some faster than others. You both only give your mum another seventy-five years or so. But her saying it out loud means it is happening faster, not slower.

You're a doctor, and there'd been warning signs big enough to see from space. She'd switched from popping pills at home to weekly chemo in the hospital, hooked up to the meds, sitting in a deep chair like a throne. Her skin was polished smooth of hair. Her lungs were being regularly drained of fluid.

I'm dying, she says.

She's dying. It's like the countdown on a bomb. She knows that. She's always had a flair for the dramatic that explodes out of her at inopportune moments with the heady exhilaration of a wine glass smashed into an ex's face. Bubbling out and burning like porridge from a pot. She doesn't even need a drink to release it, it's always there.

When you were kids you used to goad her about wanting attention. You accused her of performing for the grown-ups at dinner parties, you said they wheeled her out for entertainment like a belled monkey at a circus. You used that phrase. You were seven years old, and you even wrote it in your diary. She was eleven, and thumped you over the head with her textbooks, and wrote in her own diary, gleefully, that she had hit you and you had cried.

She showed you the entry with pride when you were friends again. 'Roopa cried BUCKETS!'

Friend is too big and small a word for what you were. You had shared a long, thin room, a divide across the middle like a belt. She got the window and the record player and you got the door and the bookshelves. You were generous with physical affection and violence.

Long childish cuddles on the sofa. Casual childish slaps and scratches and kicks and punches. You told her she'd go to jail if she were a man, for hitting you the way she did. You said she'd hit someone else when she was grown-up and really go to jail, and she was so upset you had to hug her better.

And you both want to laugh, again, inappropriately. But she's dying.

She has that smile. Those eyes. That direct gaze.

Yes, you reply, smiling back. Yes. You've got my attention. Yes, I'm chill. This moment, this everything. It's all about you.

How long? you ask. That countdown. Years, months, weeks, days, tomorrow, today, teatime, now.

Christmas, she says, an apologetic shrug.

You know what she means. Why do people always say things like that? Things like, She might make it through Christmas.

We're Muslim. Christmas just means buying more plastic crap for the kids and trying to work through the mince pies that our mum has bulk-bought. Christmas doesn't mean shit.

Except that from today, this day of kitchen table dying declarations, Christmas is less than twelve weeks away.

You both know that even death won't change the plastic crap for the kids, or the mince pies. Maybe death doesn't change everything as much as love. The pouring of endless tea, that sharing of fruit cake, these deep tyre tracks of tradition are ground into our soil.

You're not sure it's a comfort to know how little things will change when we pass, that we won't leave a mark that wasn't already there. You'll be angry later, so angry, at how quickly she dissolves, when it's over. When her small body is gift-wrapped for God, in blank white cloth, boxed up and buried under great clots of mud. Ripples slipping away in flattening circles, leaving the pond still and frozen.

You thought you'd both have more time. Fuck knows what you thought you'd do with it. Ten years came and went and for a long while she was clear and cancer-free and then suddenly she wasn't, and you're sure she spent most of that time being vaguely pissed off with you for being you. You're pissed off with you now for the same reason.

You're still smiling like you can't help it, you must look insane. You can't help it, like a skin-stripped skull can't help it.

You spoke to one of the consultants in your hospital who has the death talk every Friday, when patients come in for their test results. The clinic is for patients on the urgent cancer two-week pathway. Sometimes the results of the investigations are definitive.

Thumbs up. Thumbs down.

It's going to be all right. It's going to be as bad as it could possibly be.

Nobody wants miserable people around them when they're dying, the consultant said. It's enough to deal with already, without having to cope with everyone else being sad. It's not their fault they're dying.

You get that. You remember the lesson. Don't make your grief her responsibility. It's not about you.

So you smile, and she smiles back. Just to show what a good sister you are, that she is. You can measure it by the inch-width of the smiles.

You're not important to her right now. So you let her know that she's the most important person to you. Right here and now. You give her that.

Maybe she thinks it's a shame she had to die for this to happen. This recognition. Some people get it given to them on a plate their whole lives.

You're staring out of her wall of French windows, desperately looking for something to say. Her garden looks nice, but it always looks nice, because she pays someone to keep it that way. The conversation plays out in your head, Garden's looking good. Yes, she'd say, I might be dying, but at least I had a nice garden. There's an indeterminate brown bird hopping near the borders. Oh look, there's a bird, you could say, and when she turns to look at it you could escape and leave your chair spinning behind you.

You think of the fox you passed on the way to work the day before, lying in the fields next to the path, plumply soaking up the sun. Soft and ginger against the spiky green weeds. So tame it didn't even twitch when you walked right by it. You think you could tell her about the fox, about your long commute strolling along the field, but then it sounds like you've finished talking about her and are already talking about you.

Garden, bird, fields, fox. Like a bucolic painting. A scene from *A Room with a View*. The silence is sunlit, bright and blinding.

Let's go to Florence, you blurt out, stupidly. And once you've said it, you mean it. Why not Florence? She loved *A Room with a View*. And she'd said it was her favourite city she visited on her last longish trip. Her memory-making sick-kid-to-Disneyland tour of Europe. She messaged you the views from trains flying on rails over ravines and rolling past mountains. She messaged you from posh restaurants, posing with a wine glass. The wine glass was always full, probably poured for the photo. She barely drank.

I'm not going to Florence again, she says. She answers the why-not before you say it.

I'm not going anywhere again.

Her lungs are pretty fucked and she needs a wheelchair for long trips and a cane for the tube.

She's not expecting a Florentine minibreak. She's not expecting a thrilling valedictory conversation. She won't die by Christmas, though, as she's stubborn as hell. She's around long after Christmas.

But that won't make this a story with a happy ending.

That fox you saw lying in the sun. He was there the next day, and the day after that. It took you a while to admit to yourself that he wasn't sleeping in the sun. He was dead. The season changed, it became cool and then it became frosty, and the fox was draped in silver frost every morning, like a fairy cape.

The last possession she has is your mother's scarf, wrapped around her minutes after she passed away. Your mum was worried that she looked cold.

You're given back your mother's scarf when they cut the clothes from her body, on the day of her funeral. They unwind it gently and pass it to you, and you don't know what to do with it.

Your mother doesn't want it back. She tells you to keep it. It's nothing special, she says, just something she happened to be wearing on the bus, on the way to see your sister. But just like that, the scarf has suddenly become a holy relic and emblematic of something you cannot explain. You stuff the scarf in your bag; it still smells of your mother's perfume, of your sister's cold storage, of something chemical and creepy. You keep it, because there is nothing else you can do.

Throughout her last days of illness, you're always hoping, in that drowsy hospice, for something smaller than her previous life. The bar is low. You are hoping that she'll wake just a little, flicker open her eyes. You're hoping that she'll sip a little, from the cup held to her lips. Say a little, say hello, goodbye or just hi, or bye. Smile a little, when she hears her mother, her children.

You don't hope for anything as outrageous as her frank gaze, a spoon raised to her open mouth, a conversation or a laugh.

How quickly we settle for less.

She used to find your no-filter confessionals somewhere between amusing and pathological. People don't want to know, she said. They don't need to know every single thing that you're thinking or doing or saying. They don't want to know if your marriage is in the shitter, that you've lost all the skin off your tits.

You'd written about marriage counselling, and about eczema, for the broadsheets and the glossy mags. She didn't mind coming across it in the paper on a cafe table, or waiting at the dentist. She just didn't want you talking about it.

And anyway, she didn't say those exact words. Shitter and tits weren't in her vocabulary. But the gist. You're trying to hold on to someone so they don't just become a smudge of a symmetrical face in a smart dress, and a silhouette of a haircut. But they're gone. And you blaspheme by imagining, and then they're just another part of you. In your head, in your body. Like you inhaled and digested her.

You never promised not to write about her. And she never asked you not to do that. She knows what you're like. It's in your nature. Like the scorpion who asks the frog for the lift across the river, and stings her before they reach the opposite bank, so they both drown.

Why did you do that? she asks helplessly, as her limbs are paralysed, as she sinks beside you.

I can't help it, replies the scorpion. It's in my nature.

You wrote her a poem and she didn't hate it. She sent it to her friends. She asked you to read it at the funeral. It was a sad poem. Achingly sincere. No gleaming-skull-smile to it. You showed, a little, that you understood the reality of this. Of her faith. She couldn't imagine being blown out like a candle. So you put her in a white spotlight instead, in the final stanza.

'My sister leads us from the dark. She steps in a circle of light.' I see you. That's what the poem really said.

You've got my full attention.

This, right here and now. It's all about you.

I

Zero Day – The Day Before Lockdown

This is happening too fast.

She only died weeks ago, and you're scribbling this in borrowed time, stolen moments in the unobserved night, like a guilty grandad sucking down a secret cigarette, a teenager staying suspiciously long in the bathroom before someone starts banging on the door. Fragments of words spat out onto the screen. Emotional vomit. Pollock on the page. You don't have the benefit of hindsight to make everything tidy and less nonsensical; you have no idea what is happening apart from the alarmist titles of unread emails and noise from social media, and you're only paying attention to what you're feeling, to what you're pushing six feet under, while you dig yourself out of bed and feed the children and march three miles to work and get on with your day.

It took you ten years to write about your dad's death, and then you wrote a whole book for him. A major publisher put it out and got it on award lists, before they realised it wasn't fiction. But actually, it was fiction, because he was all made-up, moving and shiny and distracting. Liquid mercury that filled the gaps in what was real and stable and solid. You should have called the book *The Changing Man*, but someone told you about an album by the same name, so you called it something less appropriate instead. *The Flying Man*. Suggested it on an email to your publisher and that was it. You make decisions too lightly.

Big decisions, small decisions.

Big decisions like whether to marry someone. You were asked on your third date, and it wasn't even a particularly good one. You went along with it, as someone else's fierce certainty is too compelling to fight.

Big decisions like whether to leave your job and move abroad. And live out of a car and a bag.

Big decisions like whether to buy a wrecked money pit in a foreign field. Showering from a plastic bottle hung on a cherry tree in the sunlight. A watering can nozzle taped on as a shower head.

Big decisions like whether to have fertility treatment for a baby. While you're still in marriage counselling. For that relationship you tumbled into when you were nineteen. A relationship in which you were literally camping between the tent in a foreign field and your £200 car. You're still unsure if you were both just too lazy to leave.

Big decisions like whether to train in medicine. Walking to the interview in borrowed shoes, thinking, are they really going to let you do this? A thirty-something dilettante, back from abroad with four kids and an irrelevant degree. They're nuts. It's on them if they let you in. Not you.

You came in the top 3 per cent in the country in the graduate medical entrance exam. You'd home-studied biology and chemistry and physics books you took out of the library. You scored top nationally in the essay paper, but to be fair, you were probably the only published novelist among the ten thousand applicants sitting the exam in football-pitch-sized rooms around the major cities.

Top 3 per cent in the country, and you didn't suck at interview, although you nervously shook hands so long and enthusiastically with each interviewer that it must have looked like you just wanted a grown-up's hand to cling on to. You were never this anxious as a child. Still, anxiety is more appealing than confidence. It must be. They let you in.

Their certainty.

Your guilt.

On the first day of medical school, you dressed like you'd never dress again in that place. A fitted frock with statement flowers larger than both your hands, the same outfit you wore for a women's magazine prize-giving.

You asked the first question in a vast lecture room filled with hundreds of students. You sat in a group in a pub with future friends, and wandered around the Freshers' Fair with them, collecting freebies like it was a strategic scavenger hunt. You sat in another lecture room crammed with gossiping new medics making connections, and then the senior years came in and one Year Rep was a bit of a dick, and the less dick-ish one whooped, Aren't you excited! You're all going to be doctors! There was an embarrassed, faux-ironic cheer. Smiles all round. Except from you.

You still didn't really believe it.

She was convinced that you only decided to be a doctor because she was a lawyer. Doctor beats lawyer, right? Everything beats tent-dwelling dilettante writer.

You didn't tell her the truth, in case it upset her. You hadn't even been thinking about her at all. It was never a competition for you. Never is. You stroll through your story, gathering the points and plaudits lightly like flowers in a field, and dropping them just as easily. Or they fall from you, preferring the path to your possession. Praise and shame don't weigh you down.

You're glad of that.

Praise, especially, dissolves like rain on the sea and you're invisible and unheard, and nobody really knows who you are, and sometimes it feels like you could do or say anything and it would never be remarked upon.

Unless someone was seeking you out to find something to resent.

Despite books and TV appearances and double-page spreads in the broadsheets and tabloids and glossy magazines, despite the shiny photo shoots, you can still count anonymity as your achievement.

No trolls. No embarrassment. No digging.

You're glad of that too. When you were little, you always said Chris Lowe of the Pet Shop Boys was the most successful pop star. Because he could take off his hat and glasses and be like anyone else.

It's not that things come easily to you, but maybe that's how it looks. You make the big decisions too lightly, but then you stick to them stubbornly, refusing to leave something unfinished.

A proposal on a drunken third date becomes a twenty-five-year marriage.

A fertility appointment becomes four kids.

An online application form becomes a place at medical school.

And even an unmarked CD in your dad's suitcase, which was meant to have his autobiography but was actually blank, becomes your own four-hundred-page award-nominated novel.

You don't stop what you start. You don't press pause. So you just add another ball and keep on juggling.

Mother, mother, mother, mother.

Book, book, book, book, book, book, book.

Lecturer, tutor, teacher, fellow. Medical student. Junior doctor.

Like the funfair on the beach.

Scream if you want to go faster.

You're not surprised you pissed her off.

You washed her body in scented water, wrapped her in plain white cloth. Her face was uncovered until everyone had said goodbye, and then you refolded her face in the pleated cloth like a flower closing petals against the night.

It was all about her, and now suddenly, it's not. And it's not about you, either. Something else is happening.

And it's all happening too fast.

In the few weeks since she's died, the world has changed.

You're back at work two days after the funeral. It feels you're always working and always tired, and you're grateful to the hospital for not giving you time to think for the whole length of your shift. You eat your lunch one-handed, standing up at a rolling computer which you wheel about the ward, while you look up blood results, order investigations and imaging, draft patient referrals and discharge papers.

In the sad fog, in the painful aftermath of her body being awkwardly lowered into the coffin and then into the ground, you are not paying attention to the news. You hear some background noise, people are complaining about Harry and Meghan moving house to another country, you suppose it's the one where she has her roots, although you're not interested enough to ask the question. The scandal is that they didn't tell the Queen, or they did but after they told everyone else, and you're baffled at how this is the headline news. How this is what gets through.

Grandson doesn't tell Gran he's moving country, but his wife blogs it.

Amid the moral outrage that anyone would dare move to a less judgemental country with a less intrusive and injured press, there's some mention of a new virus that doesn't sound as bad as Ebola or Influenza A. The name is quite pretty, Coronavirus, and the space-alien image of the virus is quite pretty too, it sort of has a crown if you squint a lot and someone has already told you to look for it. When you first hear about Coronavirus you dismiss it. Yes, it's all very sad, and it sounds like another swine flu, or bird flu, or something to do with bats, with animal vectors, somewhere far, far away.

You see the cheerful market footage in China, the sale of livestock, of pigs, birds, bats, and you think, that's there, and this is here.

People are getting off planes from China every day, and you dismiss that. You denounce anyone talking about avoiding Chinatown in Soho as bigots. You roll your eyes at people wearing masks, the same ineffectual mask all day, as you've been taught they're single-use only, to be changed after a single interaction with a single other person.

When you hear what is really happening in China, not delightful daily markets, but the silencing of the whistle-blowers, you start to pay it some attention.

It turns out that people transmit the virus through fairly casual contact; animals aren't vectors at all, except as surfaces. You don't have to share a needle. You could be sharing an outdoor table.

Maybe someone told you why it was called Covid-19, but you've forgotten. Maybe it's the nineteenth Coronavirus, or maybe it was isolated in 2019. You're embarrassed you don't know, but not bothered enough to spend two minutes googling it.

When you see what is happening in Italy, you didn't feel as fearful as you should. Like everyone, you share the funny videos of Italian mayors berating those who were breaking the lockdown.

'You want a party at home? Have the party, and I'll send around the police with flamethrowers!'

'Why are you playing table tennis outside? Go home and play video games, you idiots!'

Idiota! Lo Stupido! You're not sure that's what they're really saying, above the subtitles, but whatever they're saying sounds better in Italian.

All the LOLs, people reply. LMFAO.

When a colleague of Chinese origin clears his tube carriage by sneezing during rush hour, you think he's right to be offended.

When an elderly lady squawks in a cafe, Are there any Italians here? before she sits down, you think she's an old bigot. You live in a town that's full of foreign students taking English classes in a college by the beach. They come from all over Europe and Asia, sent by wealthy parents who can afford this sort of thing.

You're still thinking, it couldn't happen here.

There are cases all over London, scattered cases in Oxford, some cases in your hospital, before you stop hugging people hello and goodbye. There are 130 deaths in the country before you stop shaking hands. You're two weeks behind Italy, and still no one is talking about lockdown. Literary parties are still held. Colleagues still go for Friday night drinks. You join them. You stand in crowds with cocktails.

The prime minister announces proudly that he shakes hands with everybody in a hospital photo op, including those with Covid. The medical type beside him tries to imply that he washed his hands in-between, but no one believes that.

The deaths in Italy. The mournful footage of people singing opera from their balconies. It's meant to be heart-warming, but it just makes you think of hostages at an embassy party, coming dressed-up to a place for wine and laughter and canapés, and then finding that they can never leave, and if they did, there would be nowhere for them to go.

You cancel out-of-town meetings. You stop taking trains and tubes. You keep your distance.

You say apologetically that it's because you're a doctor, and you have a duty of care for your patients. You know that non-medical colleagues think you're being precious.

The US president describes it as the Chinese virus. Some fans defend this online. It is Chinese, they argue, it came from China.

You came from your mum's vagina, comes a snappy reply, we call you Steve.

Medical colleagues are on their phones in A&E, while you're on the hot take. The front-door admissions. Doctors senior to you squashed in the tiny doctor's office. Registrars and consultants. It's not worth the risk, they say, to spouses and siblings and parents.

They're pulling their children out of schools. Ask if you're doing that too.

You do not. You've done some research, and it seems that children are invincible. Mild symptoms or nothing at all, says one ITU consultant in London. Maybe they're asymptomatic carriers. Maybe these smiling, safe children are granny-killers, but no one really knows. You're shocked at how little everyone knows. Senior medical consultants are asking if anyone knows how they can get tested, whether they should be buying hydroxychloroquine from the Indian internet. They say that's what the American president is taking.

You carry on doing your job.

Without really realising it, you've been working on the frontline of the Covid-19 crisis. It started over February, it has accelerated over March. You're doing the same job you've always done, but the language about it is changing. Frontline. It's a Battle. Doctors are described as Soldiers, patients are described as Fighters. We Can Beat It, they say. She Beat it. She's a Covid Survivor.

It's a war.

You haven't taken any of that in. It's just a few weeks since she died, and you go to work to forget. There was just one day you didn't go to work, the day after her funeral. You did go in actually, but they looked at you in shock when you arrived on the ward.

Go home, they said, just go home.

You hadn't realised you'd looked like that. You'd brushed your hair and worn a dress, but they still saw something you didn't, and sent you back.

So you just sat at home writing needy tweets to the universe about her death that slowly went viral, and you could see her rolling her eyes and mouthing in exasperation, It's STILL not about you.

It's not about you.

It's about the dying and the dead. And they are now legion. It only took a few days. Still no lockdown. People are being discharged daily with their coughs and sneezes and unremarkable diseases, back to their families, their community, their care homes, unsuspicious and unsuspected. Still no testing. People crowding out the public parks in nice weather. The advice was to stay safe and distant.

Footage of people complaining about people doing something that they themselves are doing becomes a meme.

Look at all these people on the grass, says the person filming on the grass.

You are all so stupid. You all think it couldn't happen here. As though sheer force of will and indignation could make it so.

It's happening here, but we don't accept what we do not want. Liberty is costing lives.

You're meant to be trained in the Respirator Fit testing, with the FFP2 mask tight and waterproof, like goggles, and the hood. For personal protection. You'd received emails to go and get it done on the respiratory ward, at a certain hour on a certain day, but each time you'd arrived, they didn't seem to know too much about it and said it was probably happening on a different day, or a different week. And then they said they weren't doing it anymore. Except for special cases. You're not sure why. The night registrar turns up with a certificate, having been tested. He'd got the respiratory consultant who heads up Internal Medicine to approve it.

I'm on A&E this weekend, you say, isn't that a special case?

It isn't.

During a quiet moment on your on-call, between discharging one patient and waiting for another, you go to the Intensive Care Unit, and find one of the sisters there who's been training the intensivist teams with the special masks. She trains you then and there, showing you how to put on the mask and how to check it is working. She sprays a foul smell in the air, and the test is that you can't detect it. She does this as a favour, as you used to work on ITU. You don't know how anyone else got it done. It doesn't matter, as the rules change. You don't have to be fit-tested to wear the most appropriate mask to protect yourself.

You're admitting and assessing suspected patients in A&E. You're not wearing any protective equipment, apart from the usual gloves which are worn for procedures. You're not even in full scrubs, as there aren't any trousers in your size.

This doesn't bother you, as it doesn't bother anyone. You all think that the Covid patients are special cases, known about and already isolated, and you don't think of the virus as swimming about the people around you. You do what your med reg and senior house officer are doing with the on-call medical take. You listen to the patient's concerns and examine them, noting their cough and breathlessness. Reviewing their chest X-ray and scrolling through their blood results for low lymphocytes and raised inflammatory markers. If a patient has another reason for their coughs, wheezes, sneezes, temperature, your medical registrar tells you they are probably low risk, and they don't even get swabbed. Most people have a reason. Past history of asthma, or COPD (chronic obstructive pulmonary disease) from long-term smoking, or hay fever, or another disease, or another treatment. One patient has neutropenic sepsis from her chemotherapy for breast cancer with lung metastases. Low risk. Despite her plummeting blood pressure and low neutrophils.

You work out her low risk by asking and answering these questions.

Fever? Myalgia? Cough? Chest X-ray changes? Anosmia? Foreign travel? Contact with someone with Covid?

Your medical registrar assures you that No to all of these means Low Risk.

To others at least. Not great for her, a chemo patient, like your sister was, to be in a hospital with an immune system ravaged and rebelling like that.

The low-risk patients are placed in the bay, with up to five other patients, with Health Care Assistants taking their observations, their heart rate, respiratory rate, temperature, blood pressure, oxygen saturations, with nurses coming close to administer medication. Contact is unavoidable and is offered with kindness, a reassuring hand while a needle goes in, while pills are offered and fluids set up.

You perform a bedside examination, percussing the lungs, listening to bases, feeling along the spine for bony metastases.

You wash your hands and go to another bay.

The nurse washes her hands, and goes to the next patient on her drug round.

By the end of your shift, you're told that one of your patients is now suspected Covid positive. It turns out she wasn't low risk after all. She's moved to isolation.

This is what you all do, all the time. None of you think it is unsafe. None of you think you are heroes. None of you think you are soldiers, dodging spinning bullets shaped like pretty viral crowns.

You don't feel fearful, as you don't know the risks. The virus is insidious and the background noise of the news is too garbled for your full acknowledgement.

On your long weekend in A&E, you're more concerned about missing Mother's Day because you're working a thirteen-hour shift. You see the cards propped up on the sofa when you get home late, hours after they are all in bed. The picture your daughter drew of you flies around the internet. You wanted to share it as you love the deep, dark shade of the pen she chose, that she coloured in your whole face with a bold, brown scribble. Mothering Sunday, and you only saw them for an hour in the morning. You hate how you obsess over your working-mother guilt.

You're home the next day, anyway. It's zero day. Technically a zero-hours day, your Monday off from the hospital, after three days of thirteen-hour shifts across the weekend. You are spending it supervising Oxford masters students on feminist fairy tale and conspiracy-led dystopia. In between the Skype and online supervisions and workshops, you mark graduate essays and cook salmon with garlic and turmeric, and chop vegetables and fruit for the children.

That evening, you nit-check them and cut their hair, as lockdown has finally been announced, and there won't be any hairdressers for a few months, and no one to see if you've done a bad job. You do a good job. You cut your eldest son's hair back to his shoulders. You crop your second son's hair everywhere, the way he prefers it, and curve it clearly around his precise little ears, and you shave angles into his sideburns.

This is your zero day. Everyone's zero day, as the count starts from now. Lockdown day 1 will be tomorrow, and should feel like a bigger moment, but instead it just dissolves into a list of things to do and not to do, and it feels like something inevitable and unremarkable, like a cold night following a cool day. The prime minister waving his hands around to a front-facing camera like an old-fashioned fascist feels unremarkable too. It's background noise while you are doing something with the kids.

The journalists say that you're doing the most feared job in the country. It doesn't feel like it on your day off, while you are marking papers, teaching graduates, cooking salmon, removing nits, cutting hair.

You touch your children with the same hands that were touching the patients in Emergency who are now suspected positive for Covid-19. You gently blow the hair from their necks. You tug the metal comb from scalp to tip.

2

Their Stories

The next day, the first day of lockdown, you will be back at the hospital, while everyone else stays at home. You will do this dance again for your patients. Holding their wrists to feel their pulse. Listening to their heart beat. Listening to their lungs for air entry down to the bases. Equal or unequal. Crackles or clear. You do a full physical examination of each patient. Feeling their stomach for tension and tenderness, for oversized organs of chronic disease. Pulling at their arms and legs and hands and feet for muscle weakness and neurological signs, looking into their eyes and mouths. Examining their skin.

Listening to their story, while they cough and sputter.

Each patient tells a story. It is written on their body when they don't have the words to share.

Sometimes it's banal.

She's got a bit of seasonal allergies. A bit of trouble with her asthma.

Sometimes it is brutal.

He's got a raging fever. He's had a cough for years from lung cancer. He's had surgery and chemotherapy and now it's palliative. He has no detectable lymphocytes.

He goes into isolation, and then to the respiratory ward, to the closed bay. Dying slower, dying faster. He's got what your sister had. Chemo and then an infection. Lungs soaked in fluid. You can see the signs from space.

You are inches from him as you listen to his chest.

On the first day of lockdown you get home at 10 p.m., after walking an hour along the empty dual carriageway, along the cabbage and cauliflower fields. You're relieved that it's too dark to see the ragged body of the fox, decaying just off the path's edge. You're developing a creepy fascination with it, you think of taking a photo of it daily, and watching it crumble to dust in stop-motion. You could call it After Life and offer it as modern art to a local gallery. A forensic examination of mortality and memory, the little white card would say.

You check on the sleeping children upstairs in your home. You hunt around for tooth fairy money, for gold pound coins that you can slip under their pillows.

They still believe in fairies. They reason there's no point in not believing in them, as then the fairies will cease to come. Their hair looks pretty good.

You're good with your hands, for someone so comically clumsy in everyday life, spilling drinks and tripping over pavement cracks. Once you stepped on a garden rake like Sideshow Bob.

When you stitch in a central line at a patient's throat, holding the line in place, which you slide straight through to the heart, down the jugular vein, you do it neatly, four parallel sutures, tying the surgical hand knots so fast it looks like a magic trick to those who haven't yet learned how to do it.

When they're all in bed you don't have a drink. You start writing this, instead. No one really knows what you do. Your colleagues at work know nothing of your other life at home, your other life in literature. Your family and friends and literary colleagues only have a vague idea of what doctors do, based on showboating TV that both overplays your roles and underestimates your graft.

Anyway, if you told them, no one would believe you.

Your worlds collide in your head, in your dreams. An essay on the female form used in literature for pleasure and violence. A woman lying stiff and cold in the morgue, under an ice-damp sheet, as you examine her ahead of cremation to complete her death certification. The kaleidoscope of domestic tasks scattering and reforming and never completed. You're painfully aware of doing the bare minimum in everything, and especially this last. You can handle complicated clinical procedures and difficult professorial duties, but you struggle to provide clean plates, clean clothes, hot food and fresh fruit. You struggle to keep order at home without resentment or raising your voice.

The patients in the hospital arriving, healing, dying, leaving through the front door, or boxed up and rolling out the back. All these kites, flying in the air. All these lives, unfurling and overlapping in the same day.

You know this isn't normal, but you are now unsure how normal women and men make it through each day, without all these lives shouting for attention.

You're so very special, someone once sang to you in a club when you were a teenager. You'd rejected him, and it took you a long time to realise that it wasn't a compliment. Your sister said something similar, years later. She said, It Must Be Great To Be You, and you heard the sharpened point to her words.

You put fresh yellow daffodils on the corner of the table that you've set aside for her sympathy cards. The first flowers you had received after her death have dried elegantly in the vase. You can't bring yourself to clear it all away. No one else will touch it, the little makeshift shrine.

The most feared job in the country.

Feminist fairy tale. Conspiracy dystopia.

Haircuts.

Nits.

Pandemic

Lockdown.

There's a lot going on.

How many times have you all lived through the fearful and extraordinary, and felt that everything was irrelevant?

On 9/11 you watched the footage at work. You went home, because you were sent home. Your office was too near the American Embassy. You watched *Bridget Jones*, ate a takeaway and probably had sensible sex afterwards.

When the bus exploded in London, you were in another part of town. When the brown guy was shot on the tube, you stopped carrying a backpack to work. And you never ran on public transport again. When Grenfell burned, you were living in a semi near the beach. You used to live near Grenfell; you probably walked past it with friends after school, heading into Kensington. You don't live near anywhere anymore.

Nothing touches you. Nothing is important. Nothing you do is important. And now.

You're in the eye of the storm. It's quiet and still. The news reports your work, and that of your colleagues, as extraordinary. But routine makes it banal. So you touch the people no one wants to touch. So you prescribe them banana-flavour protein drinks to build up their cachectic frames. Or chocolate. Or mocha for a treat. You try to be kind. You try to do no harm. They say you are risking your life. Risking your family. Risking everything.

It doesn't feel like that.

Maybe it's not that everything is irrelevant. Maybe it's just that you are. It feels like a relief to say that out loud.

It's Not That Great To Be You.

You wish your sister were there to hear it. She was stubborn, and so are you. You say it to her anyway. You keep her there, at her place laid at your kitchen table, and she'd probably rather be anywhere else. She didn't like where you lived. The beach, the sky, the good state schools. It was all too careless, it was all about showing her up.

She was always telling you to leave the house on the coast, saying it took you too far from the family. She blamed your partner, and told you to leave him, too.

As though leaving is so easy.

Why does Auntie live down here? your niece asked her, on a rare visit. Your twins' first birthday. Because she's poor, she snapped.

You glared at each other. And then you laughed. Conspirators, again. It was actually quite funny. Her timing was good. She knew how to deliver a line, and you never told her how much you admired that about her.

Maybe it's the end of the fucking world as we know it. As if we ever knew it. Maybe her death wasn't the terrible tragedy you made it out to be. Maybe she just beat the queue.

Happy Birthday, you say to her. You're writing her a card.

She decided she was going to live forever. She went god-squad, so it's her fault, not yours, that she's sticking around. You send a picture of the daffodils to your mum. Yellow. Impertinent. Stiff.

Her birthday isn't today, the day you're writing the card. It's in a couple of days.

You see, you tell her, I haven't forgotten. If I sent this card tomorrow, you'd get it in time.

You remembered her birthday. She used to forget yours on purpose. Make it a point of pride. Aren't you too OLD for birthdays, she'd say, weeks later. Promising to post you something or take you somewhere, and you both knew it would never happen. You'd promise the same imaginary thing for her birthday, to make it even.

Well, then, we might as well just get it for ourselves, she'd say, and you'd agree. It was uncertain who won and lost at these little imaginary transactions.

She'd been saying you were too old for birthdays since your teens.

You're not going to send the card. Not to her home address, to the house where her husband and children live, a place that's been emptied of her. That would be psychotic.

You tuck it in with the other condolence cards on the table. No one will see that you did this apart from her.

You see her rolling her eyes at you. Well, now you're just showing off.

3
Healers and Hitch-hikers

It's the second day of lockdown. It's the second day of home-school, of home-everything, unless you're a key worker. The newsfeeds state that 422 people are dead in the UK from Covid-19. India is in lockdown too. One fifth of the planet. The future king has the virus. Mildly. An Oscar-winning actor is recovering from it. A bit smugly.

The virus has a lack of respect for the traditional boundaries of privilege. Despite the US president describing it as the Chinese virus, it swims everywhere, on our breath and dives into the depths of our lungs, it slides on surfaces and waits for a host, patiently, for days.

A hitch-hiker by the roadside with a knife in his backpack.

He's tolerated by children. He taunts healthy adults. He torments and tortures the old and sick.

Most successful viruses don't kill their host, as if they did, they couldn't keep going around. Like the scorpion riding the frog across the river, it's of no benefit to sting her; they'll just go down together. So he doesn't really want to kill you, but sometimes he just can't help it.

It's in his nature.

She's not fit for ventilation. You hear that all the time. In the beginning, it is said with apologetic explanation. Then it just feels like a flat No. Not for Ventilation. Not a candidate.

Like getting into the Intensive Care Unit is like getting into some exclusive club, and she didn't make the cut.

It is and she didn't.

A failing, ageing body wouldn't survive the interventions that a younger body would shrug off in moments. Sedation. Intubation. Ventilation.

Someone told you that you weren't meant to be alive past forty, in evolutionary terms, and every moment afterwards is borrowed.

Borrowed from what? Some future life? Some better life? Some party happening downstairs, and you're still deciding whether to wander down and join in.

That sounds just as terrifying. Who really likes parties? If you liked them, you wouldn't need to be drunk to enjoy them.

You saw some people bouncing around your sister's funeral like it really was a party. Every eye dry. Every drink dry as well. Now that she'd decided to out herself as religious. She'd never worn a hijab in her life, but all her friends and family had to wear one for her mosque prayers. Some wore it casually, a Grace Kelly type scarf lightly draped over their hair. Some wore it properly, neatly tucked in and obviously advised on the pinning by more observant friends.

People didn't recognise you until you removed yours. Your own mother didn't recognise you, and you were wearing the scarf she'd loaned to you, dark blue with pale birds, like doves.

Your face is anyone's face, really, you have two of those eyes and one of those mouths, and your face is only really defined by the curve of your eyebrows and shape of your hair. People used to mistake you for other people with the same hair all the time. You can't be caricatured, as you have nothing that distinguishes you. Your cartoon is just a haircut and a smudge of a face beneath a fringe. You could be invisible, if you wanted. And you did want to be, at her funeral. Watching those people work the room, laughing, chatting and catching up. Actually saying, with a hug, with a laugh, We must get together soon around my place.

They were so shiny and smiley. Psychopaths. You hoped they got eaten by their cats.

You don't why you're writing this. You told yourself you'd never write again. You don't know why you thought you were so special, as though the world needed another one of your books on the shelf.

And the world really doesn't want another book from another eccentric middle-class novelist. You don't have to look like Mrs Woolf, to be thin and white, to be in a place of privilege, too.

And yet you're writing, because like she said, you have this urge to confess. You write because you must. It's really like a disease. And you think of all the hundreds of thousands of words of confession you wrote, and no one really noticed, because you wrapped it up in fiction and pretended it was anyone but you.

Six books published, six unpublished. Two published for children. Four unpublished for children. Stories of being a daughter, a wife, a mother, a sister. You call yourself a storyteller. But you're not. None of it was a story. You're not a good liar. Everything was true.

4

Birthday

Today. It's her birthday, today. Your family had planned a big celebration of her life to be held on her birthday, with all her friends, maybe in her garden, maybe in a local hall. A proper event, with pictures and food and music, where your children could attend and hide under tables with snacks and devices. The funeral had been rushed as Muslim funerals must be, for the dead to be buried as soon as the mosque could arrange it, and not everyone who cared about her could attend at short notice.

She had already curated a playlist for the event, being as organised as she was stubborn. That's a nice way of saying controlling. You have to be nice about the dead. It was going to be all about her. There was going to be a reading of the poem you wrote about her, at her request. There would definitely be cake.

The event is cancelled. Indefinitely postponed like everything else.

Today you should have been reading a poem, and eating cake with family, and being kind to elderly acquaintances, and maybe you would have expiated your judgement of people who bounce about at funerals like parties. Maybe they just don't get out much and were genuinely pleased to see distant relatives and old friends. Maybe this alternate version of you is chatting to them, right now.

You don't have time to think about the ghost non-event in the non-Covid reality, as you're back on shift in A&E. Thirteen hours. It's really twelve and half hours, but thirteen sounds neater when people ask you about your shift, and it's not like anyone ever leaves on time. You walk in at 9 a.m. and the rest of the hot team are fiddling with bleeps, crammed in the two-by-two-metre office, jostling for position on one of the five computers. At the handover, there are ten of you there.

The medical take team, they're all just sitting or standing there like it's a game of musical chairs in a tube carriage. Close enough to touch every other person in the room. Close enough to kiss every person in the room with just an extra step. You all know that you are meant to socially distance, but there's no possible way.

Isn't there anyone to see? you ask. You don't want to stand with them in the cramped office.

Yeah, there's this one, they say eagerly. There's an electronic board on the wall, with a patient who hasn't yet been clerked. You put your name against the patient. And find out a moment later why no one else wanted to see her. Covid-19. High Risk. Placed in the Blue Zone.

You don't ask what the Blue Zone is. Things are changing so rapidly that questioning is less helpful than simply accepting and adapting. You go down to Majors in A&E, and see it for yourself. The Blue Zone is where Minors used to be, between the front door at reception and the main section of A&E. It now has sealed doors, with staff acting as runners outside, passing essential equipment through the doors with gloved hands. It seems stuffed with medics and nurses in full PPE. Gown, gloves, visor, mask. It is where all the Covid high-risk patients have been placed.

Why's it blue, you want to ask, but it seems like a stupid question. You'd think that the danger zone would be red. Maybe it's to reassure patients, blue just sounds more calming.

Azure, Cerulean, Cyan.

Scrubs, sea and sky.

You suit up and clerk the patient along with the consultant, while your colleagues are free to look up memes in the high-risk petri-dish office.

They post ironic memes about themselves looking up memes on their private feeds.

What they say: You're an NHS Hero. (Picture of heroic doc in PPE.)

What I do: Look up memes in my office. (Picture of idiot doc smirking at his computer.)

You think your patient probably doesn't have Covid-19. She's more likely got a urine infection, and she is already fairly demented. It's an unkind adjective. It reminds you how unkind dementia is as a diagnosis, another relentless clock counting down. You arrange to move her out of the Covid-19 zone as soon as possible, but you suppose that it's possible that she's caught it while she was being triaged and treated. It's possible that you caught it too, in the Blue Zone. It's just as possible you caught it from your colleagues avoiding the Blue Zone in the squashed office space.

I think it's called the Blue Zone because it's blue for hypoxia, one of the Emergency Department nurses tells you.

Hypoxia is when you don't have enough oxygen circulating, and it causes cyanosis, demonstrated by blue lips, blue tongue, blue peripheries. Cyanosis. Cyan for Blue.

The medics are all called to a special meeting to be updated on the Covid-related changes to the rota. You go in between clerking the new patients, see the chairs neatly laid out two metres apart in the lecture theatre, and take one at the back, at the far side, so you can race out if you get an emergency bleep. You're on the hot team that covers the in-hospital medical emergencies like cardiac arrests, as well as covering the front-door incoming patients in A&E. You get bleeped for stroke calls too, as you only have a short window of time to get patients to CT scanning to check there isn't a brain bleed, and then to thrombolyse, to break down the clot that's caused the stroke. There isn't enough space, and so people hover at the back, or go to the overflow rooms and complain about the rota, or laugh at stuff on their phones, not realising that they're on camera in the main theatre, with their mics broadcasting to all rooms. It's awkward more than funny, for the people sitting with you in the lecture hall. Someone goes and tells them they're on screen, and helpfully switches off their microphones.

In the main lecture hall, during the meeting, the consultants bicker between themselves, about the lack of PPE for the non-respiratory specialities, about the cancellation of holidays for everyone until July, about how every bank holiday is gone and weekends that had been confirmed free are now back on the rotas. There's talk about getting more people redeployed into medicine and the Intensive Care Unit to help out. The surgeons have nothing to do, and almost empty wards, as all elective operations are cancelled and they're only covering emergencies.

It directly affects you, but there's nothing you can do about it. Your Easter holiday is cancelled, your half-term is cancelled, the bank holiday is cancelled, you might be redeployed into ITU to support the intensivists. You're told this without excuse or apology, and you accept that. It's not like there's anywhere for you to go, now the world has closed down. It's not like your weekend is now any different from the week, now that school is closed. For the first time in that busy day, you look at your phone. You see an explosion on WhatsApp. An outpouring of birthday messages. Her name, her photos at all ages and stages, reminiscing and recollections.

Tears start running down your face, dripping on your scrubs. Your consultant is sitting near enough to look at you questioningly. You have a different consultant each week, but this one is always kind and particularly observant. She is two metres from you, the next chair along.

You get a non-urgent bleep and use it as an excuse to leave the room, practically running out the door. Someone in the corridor asks if you are all right, and you break the accepted protocol, and give an honest answer, like a sociopath.

You even tell them why.

No, I'm not all right, you say. My sister died, and it's her birthday, and it's just hit me, and now I'm sad and can't stop crying.

You should have just said that it was your allergies. That's what you say all the time. I'm not crying, it's my allergies. I'm atopic. In the doctor world, that last phrase answers everything if you want to avoid follow-up questions. No one wants to know about someone else's hay fever.

Although it turns out, saying I'm sad and can't stop crying, that works too. You don't get follow-up questions. You get a sort of shocked disbelief that you dared to go there. It's like you slapped them. Coughed in their face with your snotty, messy tears.

Giving someone the truth when they don't want it is a sort of emotional violence. It's as much an act of aggression as shaking their hands in the Covid era.

You don't care, in that moment. You don't care that the rules are changing. Life is demonstrably too short for them.

You've already lost count of how many times people have said The New Normal. Someone has already coined Covidiot but it doesn't catch on like Brexiteer or Remoaner, maybe because everyone is meant to be on the same side.

That afternoon you see someone come up on the board when you've just become free. Elderly patient. Not too elderly. That's all you know about her. You only get a name, an age, the time she came in and the name of the ED doctor who saw her when she came in the front door. On your list because the A&E team have triaged her to medical care. That means not for the surgeons, or another speciality, like Paeds or Obs and Gynae, or Orthopaedics.

You put your name against the patient, three minutes after she was electronically handed over to you, and print out her clerking paperwork. You look her up on the hospital systems and scribble down her past medical history. A vasculopath. Diabetes, high blood pressure, on statins. You note down her usual medications, so you can chart them up. Nothing worrying, there. You see that bloods were taken when she came into ED, and check if the results are here. They've started coming in.

The numbers are terrifying. Kidneys are shut down, with creatinine sky-high. The liver function tests show that hepatocytes, the liver cells, have been killed off in huge numbers. The troponin, the cardiac measure, is a few thousand above the highest you've ever seen. This patient is in multi-organ failure. Probably after a myocardial infarction. A heart attack that might have been missed. In danger of another arrest, any time.

You gather the papers and see the notes coming in from ED. A nurse has seen her now to take her observations, and these are terrifying too. Her ECG is pre-arrest rhythm. She's just been cardioverted by the locum ED consultant you saw that morning.

This was a consultant who held out his hand to you decisively when you introduced yourself, and you stared at him and his ungloved hand like he was a moron or like you were. You're still not sure if it was some sort of test.

The patient is on oxygen, working hard to breathe. She's in the Resus bay, with a kindly nurse looking after her. You talk to her, examine her, interpret her next ECG, which looks like she's had a heart attack. But she still hasn't been started on the ACS protocol by the Cardio reg who looked at the ECG, or by the ED consultant.

You start intravenous fluid for the acute kidney injury; it seems that they've shut down altogether. She's only produced 7ml of urine in the time she's been in the hospital. You make sure the bag of fluid is warm, as she came in hypothermic, and that will help heat her up. You start calcium resonium as her potassium has shot up, which could cause another arrest. You ask the consultant why she hasn't been started on ACS protocol, for acute coronary syndrome, and they say the Cardiology reg thought she had fast atrial fibrillation, not a heart attack.

But her troponin is 8,000, you argue. You don't think the Cardiology team realised that. The result must have come after their review.

She's been in that irregular rhythm for days, they argue back. That could have caused it.

But the T-wave inversion, you say. The Q waves.

It's like you're all speaking a foreign language that no one wants to admit they don't quite understand. However grown-up you get in medicine, maybe you never outgrow this particular failing.

Do you know what's happened? You ask the patient this gently. She is worried that she hasn't had her evening medication yet. She never misses her blood pressure tablets.

Her blood pressure meds are nephrotoxic. The tablets are fine to take if you are in good health, as controlling blood pressure is generally helpful for your kidneys, but you need to stop the tablets if you're not well and dehydrated. You think this is what's killed off her kidney function.

Just a bit poorly, she says. For a couple of days now. Just stayed in bed. But when I fell over going to the loo, my other half said I'd better go in. Had a spot of diarrhoea.

I wish you'd come in a couple of days ago, you say.

Everyone told us to stay away, she shrugs. You know, the news. I've told my husband to go home, he's very sensible, he went straight away without a fuss.

You tell her that her heart has probably been in an abnormal rhythm for the two days she's been sick. That her liver and kidneys haven't been perfused adequately because of this, and her kidneys have been shutting down, and her liver is in trouble. That she may have had a heart attack, which she didn't feel because of her diabetes, but that the diarrhoea may have been a reaction to the heart attack from the sympathetic nervous system. You tell her the truth, and say that it might happen again.

You tell her you're going to try to get a bed in Cardiology.

You tell her you're going to call the Intensive Care Unit, as if she doesn't start producing urine, she'll need haemofiltration.

Your registrar turns up, as the observations for the patient have now been posted on the online board.

Your woman's pretty sick, he says. You ask him directly if you can start the ACS protocol, but he doesn't think you should, either. The ITU team turn up, and say that there's no way they're taking up a bed for her for filtration, she's peri-arrest. It's like a death sentence.

Three days ago, before lockdown was announced, she was walking to the shops with her husband.

You chase around for the post-take consultant covering medicine. You go to the Clinical Decisions Unit, the Observations Bay, all around the shop floor, in the isolation zone. Everyone just saw him moments ago, no one knows where he is now.

You call switchboard and leave another message for him.

You're being bleeped about a stable stroke patient whom another consultant wants to see with you.

You say you're in Resus with an emergency.

You find the consultant in the Acute Medical Urgent Care Unit. You show him the ECG and say it was a heart attack, and he agrees. Your reg now decides he agrees too. You start the ACS protocol. It includes ticagrelor and aspirin. You've got a Cardiology bed.

You ask for her partner's number, and your reg calls him while you are writing up the medication and handing her over to Cardiology.

The patient still doesn't know that she's going to die. Maybe not now. But tomorrow, or the next day. Maybe the day after that.

You tell her, gently, as she gets taken to the ward. But with the cheerfulness of the nurses, the sense of going somewhere, of getting out of ED, she doesn't really take it in.

At the end of the shift, the reg says, your woman was sick. That was a terminal event.

You don't tell him how frustrated you were, that the SHO, the consultant, the other consultant, your reg all told you she hadn't had a heart attack, that you had to chase for a senior review to give the basic medication because your other seniors had said otherwise.

It wouldn't have changed anything.

She didn't have Covid-19, but the pandemic is what killed her. If she'd been able to come into A&E, or out to her GP, when she felt a bit sick, that irregular pulse would've been noticed. An ECG would have been done. She would have been shocked back to a normal rhythm two days earlier. She'd have lived with her sensible husband, and walked to the shops with him, until something else killed her instead.

We all think we have more time.

At some point in the evening, while you're on shift, people around the country step out of their front doors and clap for the NHS. It's the first time the clapping happens, and you don't know where the idea came from.

You and your colleagues on shift only found out about it later, through WhatsApp and FB messages, and little videos on Twitter.

You feel that it's a way to fake support without any cost to the clapper.

I'll take the praise, said one of the porters, working the night shift, but I'd prefer cash.

You're thinking the same, as you walk out of the hospital. It's an hour's walk along the dual carriageway to your house. You leave the car for your lockdown husband and home-schooling kids. You won't take a bus. There's no cab that would leave two metres between you and the driver, and you're the highest risk to others. You don't wear the full PPE in your ward, as you're not meant to have Covid-positive patients there, except that you do, they're just not confirmed by swab. The PPE is swept off your ward and taken to the respiratory wards with the confirmed patients.

When you get home, you shut the door behind you, and look at your messages, look at the clapping videos, reply to the messages gushing about all the love you must have felt. You feel nothing. Just numb. It's not that you're unappreciative or dead inside. It's just that it's the end of your shift.

You feel angry watching the politicians, though. Credit-grabbing feel-good photo opportunists. Led by the prime minister. Smug mop-headed bastard.

You remember what you had pushed away for hours, while you were failing to save someone's life, and just standing by, while your patient's body systems shut down.

You remember it is her birthday.

She's sitting amused on the sofa. Not lying on it like she was for the last months of her life. She's not coughing anymore. Death is great for the lungs. Her eyebrows are back, and her cropped hair is thick again. She's wearing her glasses, although she can't need them. Death has to be great for the eyes, too.

You show her the messages from her friends, from the family. Her daughter wrapped around the cherry tree they planted in her garden in her memory. The cake her husband bought for her birthday, decorated with spring flowers. They would have made one, but apparently there are no eggs in north London. You show her the photos of your mum and her partner at her grave; they had walked an hour there and then an hour back.

You write a FB message in tribute to her, listing her achievements, with her most flattering pictures. Not many people look great without hair. She's even got a stoical adolescent to smile for the selfie. Her teeth are great, too. The likes start spilling in, and she smiles. She liked being popular and never really expected it.

You need to chill, she says, it's not about you.

I'm chill, you lie. I'm perfectly chill. It's not like I cried ugly tears in public today.

Don't be sad, she says. Have cake instead.

There's no cake, but there are triple chocolate cookies you baked with your son.

She wouldn't have survived this pandemic, even if she'd been stubborn enough to survive the cancer for another couple of months.

You guess that everyone has to die of something.

I'm here, she says, I'm still right here. Sorry.

What are you doing here, you ask her. Got no mortal enemies to haunt?

Hah, she says, *Mortal* enemies. You funny.

You used to dread getting a phone call or an email from her. She was always telling you off. You used to dread the undiluted critique.

Wrong car, wrong house, wrong husband. Change it, sell it, LEAVE him.

Wrong hair, wrong dress, wrong shoes. Cut it, donate it, BIN them.

You look too old, you look too young, no one's going to take you seriously. You're too thin, you're too fat. You eat too much cake, you don't eat enough carbs.

Don't get snippy with me. I'm just trying to help.

You suppose you should have been flattered by her forensic attention. No one else looked that close. She once called you minutes after a Radio 4 interview, telling you that you were making jokes when everyone else was serious. She said, You hadn't read the room or listened before you went on, had you?

She was right. You hadn't listened, as you'd been stuck making polite small talk with your publicist over brownies in the guest green room.

So she doesn't disappoint. She tells you off.

You're still not reading the room, she says. She's talking about your FB post. No one wants a misery message. Say something funny.

Funny? You're surprised. She always kind of implied you used comedy as a crutch. Or maybe you thought that yourself.

Or at least say something true, she says. Quote a damn sonnet. You're good at quoting. You used to write Byron's stuff on the fridge when you were thirteen. All my uni friends said how pretentious you were.

OK, you say. You win, again. I'll quote something. So you add this to the message.

'Do not go to my grave and cry. / I am not there. I did not die.'

You break the cookie. Triple chocolate.

I'm just pleased you said I won, she says. 'Cause, this is, I guess, your place. You're the host. I'm the...

Virus? you scoff.

I was going to say guest, she says.

It's not pathological, you say defensively. It's perfectly normal to see the dead, for months after they die. They're in your head, all experience happens in your head. Every spike of pain, or love. Every memory.

So what happens in your head is real?

Yes.

So I'm real?

Yes.

And I won, she says.

Death perfects us, doesn't it? you say. The dead always win.

5

Scribes

It's day 7 of lockdown. You've stolen some time to write at the end of the day, but the clocks have gone back and you're too shattered and keep falling asleep at the keyboard.

There's nothing much to write, but you feel you owe a record.

To someone.

You don't know why. The record's already being kept between the news networks and Twitter. You can't stop yourself doom-scrolling once the children are in bed. You sit on the floor in the hall, your back to the radiator where their school clothes are drying, surrounded by their clutter of lunch boxes, school bags, trainers and chunky black shoes, lit by your laptop on the first stair. The kitchen and sitting room seem too cold and dark.

Three NHS doctors died from Covid-19, that's being reported today. They all have names like yours. Funny, foreign names, is what the elderly white patients say with desperate helplessness, trying to read your name badge, trying to remember the name of the other funny, foreign doctor they just saw. We all look alike to them, brown doctor, black hair, blue scrubs.

The prime minister now has the virus, and you don't know how they justified testing him for it, if he only has mild symptoms. At least the future king is elderly and met criteria.

The PM is the idiot who told the nation to take it on the chin, just a few weeks ago. Not your PM. The majority voted for him in a Boaty-McBoatface landslide of irresponsibility, because he gives good caricature. Democracy is the tyranny of the majority; that was John Stuart Mill.

It's long past midnight. You're getting up for your shift in six hours.

One of your colleagues says she's scared to come into work. You wonder why you aren't scared. You have four school-age children at home. You have so much to lose.

You can't stop yourself writing. You shouldn't write. Not unless it's something necessary that only you could write. Something with heart and meaning, which can only come from you. Like Bernie writing about Black British WomXn, Naomi and Margaret writing about Female Power.

Race and Gender. The Big Topics. What's left for you?

Your daily reality is the same as it is for everyone who works in a hospital.

Disease, Vulnerability and Death.

But now you find yourself at the frontline of an unprecedented global pandemic.

A front seat in history. Although history is always happening somewhere. We just don't pay attention to it, if it's far away, unfilmed and unreported.

This happened right here. It is forced onto every screen. It is every news report, every post and tweet. But somehow, you barely noticed it happening. You were too busy doing your job.

When a friend in Oxford didn't hug you, you thought he was being precious. When he asked you your opinion on the pandemic, citing the Italian trajectory, *la quarantena*, you thought he was being alarmist. You thought the word pandemic was overkill.

Remember when your friend of Chinese origin coughed on a tube carriage and cleared it, and you thought the escaping passengers were all bigots?

Remember when the old lady asked loudly in the cafe if anyone was Italian before she ordered, and you called her out as an old racist?

You still think they were wrong. But you were too.

And now everyone is two metres from everyone else, when they're not locked down in their homes. You suppose that everyone's writing a book, during lockdown. They're writing about isolation, about domestic violence, comic romances about mismatched couples who find themselves trapped together.

They're writing about being perched and twittering in a gilded cage, their phones providing a pocket-sized window on a wider world, while birds fly free outside. Soaring in great fluid circles over fields and seafront.

The birds own your town now. You suppose you should welcome your new feathered overlords. They're noisy chanters in the morning, but they're not doing a worse job than the last lot.

Someone clever is probably writing a version from the virus's perspective, in experimental blank verse and the first-person plural.

Doctors are too busy working to write books, even if they were the sort who wanted to write. It was a huge, humbling wake-up call that none of the doctors on your ward had heard of the Booker Prize. On medical social media, the doctors who keep a newspaper column are vilified as media-hungry opportunists. Reporting on your experiences, on patient experiences, is considered bad taste.

Those who do so are served with Who-the-hell-do-you-think-you-are?

But you're persisting in this account, to offer it to some future self who might forget. Some future other who lived through this too. The experience of disease is subjective, everyone who looks it in the face sees someone different.

Every individual experience matters, a silver thread of your own truth wound about it. You will write. A little. A lot. You can unspool this experience and share it.

Maybe, today, tonight, in these early hours, sitting in the dark of your hallway, you're the scribe for your tribe.

On this seventh day of lockdown, you get an email that four patients have died, so far, from Covid. Across the three hospitals in the Trust. Among the thousands of patients, that doesn't seem too bad. But then you read up on Twitter about those three NHS doctors who have died. There'd been talk about them in the hospital. Fearful mutinous mutterings in the mess, in the quiet corners at the ends of long corridors. The first British clinician deaths in the UK due to the virus. One is originally from Pakistan, like you. One GP, two surgeons.

The sort of people who like to say this sort of thing out loud say that they shouldn't be described as British. They're brown, from somewhere else. It doesn't matter how many times you say you're British, that questioning, where are you from, no, I mean where are you REALLY from, so where are your parents from, no, where are they REALLY from, is relentless. Comically so, almost.

The dead doctors. The brown doctors. From somewhere else, once upon a time.

You know there's no point arguing or even replying. It's like dousing a fire with petrol. But you're thinking, how much more do you have to give? When do you get to belong? A life's work devoted to caring for others. A life. Their lives. Given away.

If they had proper protective equipment, it wouldn't have happened.

How much more should they have been given? When do you get to feel safe?

You had no scrubs for your last on-call shift in A&E. You wore leggings and stole a scrub top from theatres.

They show you the Covid gear that's been issued for the Covid bay in your ward. Just a regular surgical mask and a gown. No sealed mask tested with a foul smell sprayed in the outside air, like in the training. No hood. No visor. Nothing to cover your hair, or your shoes.

You'll walk straight into the virus. You'll soak it up in your hair like a sponge. You're going to get it, too.

It's inevitable.

You're surprised you haven't got it already. You've been more exposed than anyone you know. Face to face and hand on hand with patients who have gone on to test positive.

You take that knowledge home, every night.

Every day, you walk back in the wind, along the cabbage fields. Sometimes in the sunshine, now the days are lengthening. You think that might help lift the viral load from your clothes.

You saw a photo of a single human hair studded with the virus like seeds on a strawberry.

Every day, you strip your clothes and shoes and socks as soon as you shut the front door behind you, and squash your clothes into a plastic bag and hang it high, where it can't be touched, at the entrance to the house. Your stethoscope and ID cards, which hang around your neck, have already been wiped and stuffed in a plastic packet in your handbag.

Every day, you wash your hands before you touch your children. You know how to do it properly, and you show them that you are doing it.

Every day, your hands are cracked and dry.

You hug the children, and then you dress.

They've added you to another WhatsApp group, where people complain about the viral-loaded scrubs that have been dumped in the mess, where they can infect everyone. The wards don't all have places to get the scrubs, or to put the scrubs back into the laundry cycle. It used to be just theatres and ITU who wore scrubs.

They have promised fifty sets of scrubs in the mess, which isn't enough. It's a sort of Russian roulette based on shift pattern; if you happen to be on earlies, you'll get a pair.

Today, you had bought your children the cookies you'd promised, since they had run out the last time you went shopping. Their father tried to wash the paper packets before you stopped him, as they'd be ruined if they got wet. You left them in the sun instead.

They say that the first case of coronavirus cluster in Europe was caused by someone passing the salt to someone else at a canteen, who passed it to someone else sharing their workstation, and so on and so on.

Other doctors are vocal about self-isolating from their families, but you don't even think about that. You tell yourself that children are invincible. Just as old people are vulnerable.

This is a clever, millennial virus that leans into every trope about ageing.

This is a schoolyard bully virus that stalks past the strong and spits on the weak.

You can't empathise with the online whining from clustered groups of bored people, it bothers you how they assume that every experience is their own, as they bother you with minutiae and bombard you with questions that are meant to be about you, but are really about them.

You feel pestered. Before, you only ever saw people outside the house, your place is too untidy and noisy and uncivilised to have anyone grown-up visit, but now everyone is beaming into your living room, peering out of your tablet at you, frowning over your shoulders. Distracted by your fraying at-home clothes and the clutter in the background. You still have a Christmas tree and pumpkin lanterns hanging, as the children like the fairy lights, and you suppose the season will come back around soon enough. You still have cupboards plastered with childish art and photos from Reception school projects.

Everyone sees behind the curtain. Your lecturing and charity colleagues, your friends, your mum's partner in pyjamas, your in-laws, your children's friends' parents. Judging your interiors, the Blu-Tacked pictures by the children, and withering flowers kept stubbornly on the corner of the table.

Those who don't beam in are chattering intensely and persistently on WhatsApp, even the elusive rota coordinator and administrators, popping up on your personal number, requesting your responses across weekends and evenings.

It seems inappropriate to complain. At least you're not dead. At least you're not bored.

You're back on your shift, in six hours. It feels like you only just got home.

★★★

You walk into the hospital and hunt for scrubs. Then you stride to the ward, and find a computer to start the patient list ahead of the ward round, looking through the notes of those new patients who have joined you overnight. You won't get to pee from when you start at 8.30 a.m., until after the ward round is done at 2 p.m.

You eat a sandwich with one hand while sorting out patient plans, scribbling notes and ordering tests.

You don't sit down. On principle. You're better on your feet.

You ask the ward nursing team to swab two of the long-term patients for the virus. Their observations and clinical signs are suspicious. It's not surprising if they've caught it.

Your team don't trust the negative results for patients. They say the swabs are only 70 per cent accurate, at best.

A woman is probably dying, and there's nothing they can do for her. Can't even get a line into her veins for her blood transfusions and IV replacements. She's too puffed up with fluid, and there is no visible or palpable vein.

So you get an ultrasound machine, and teach a junior how to cannulate a vein with the ultrasound screen flickering at the bedside in black and white. You show her the pulsing of the brachial artery, and how to avoid it, and the compressible vein. You unsheathe the needle, and slide it into the centre of the vein, and you see on the fluid screen the white point of the needle piercing the wall, the venous blood flowing up through the tube.

You flush sterile fluid through the cannula, before connecting it to the unit of blood hanging by the bed. The patient is relieved and thankful that you can do it at the first attempt. If you hadn't succeeded, you or someone else would have had to try and try again until it was done, as she needs her transfusions to live.

Despite all this, despite your basic competence in providing patient care, despite working fast and hard all day, working through lunch, you still leave late.

Your day is as muddled as your thoughts.

You get home and you are tempted, for a moment, not to strip at the door. Really, what's the point?

You do it anyway, as you do every-every-every day, despite feeling that you've already gone past the point of no return.

You feel the world has changed.

You saw patients' relatives stealing the hand sanitiser from the end of the bed, the same stuff that you need to keep their loved one safe. You ran out of it on the ward and were without it for a couple of hours, until someone was able to get a new supply.

You've seen shelves emptied of fruit and flour and toilet roll. Everyone has become a hermit staycationer, baking and peeing and wanking.

You feel that a crowd will be something people drool at on their screens like porn.

We'll all be dead in the next hundred years, and the ones who left early, well, they just missed the queue at the gates.

I was always punctual, comments your sister, from her place at the table, next to her withered flowers in the vase. That was one of my flaws.

It's like the set answer you practise for an interview, the acceptable weakness that shows you self-reflect. An untruth sprinkled with fairy dust. You used to say the same thing at interviews, say that you were annoyingly punctual, which was funny because it was so blatantly untrue, and un-you. Stealing her line as easily as you stepped into her smart shoes, loaned for the day because she despaired of your scruffy boots. You said it at one job interview you were thirty minutes late for, and they didn't challenge you, as they had been running too late with the other candidates to notice. You were three hours late for your Oxford interview, and missed your Economics slot with the professor. When they rescheduled, you explained inflation using the wrinkled fruit in the professor's bowl. One apple, two pears. The Economics professor told you years later that he was impressed by your use of props. By your ability to make something complex sound simple.

I was always late to the party, you reply. That's one of mine.

Not the one I'd pick, she scoffs.

6

Witness

It's day 9 of the lockdown. You don't dress smartly, as you see WhatsApp messages flying in from the hospital admin to your personal phone in a new group that they have hastily set up. (No one asked you if this was OK, this breach into your personal space, with every other junior doctor in the Trust commenting constantly in the group, like ghosts unsettled in a graveyard.) They say that there should be scrubs to wear, finally. So you'll wear leggings, and change into scrubs, and reduce by that tiny amount the virus you're bringing home to your family.

Except that when you get in, there are no scrubs delivered.

You go to the ward, explain your inappropriate wardrobe choice, and start your day.

The day starts with a complaint against you from the day before.

You were asked to write up the discharge medication urgently for a patient who was due to leave that morning. You were given less than five minutes to do it, for a harried nurse to race down to the pharmacy before it shut, so that the medications could be vetted, approved for dispensing. So the patient would be ready for her hospital transport in the morning to her specialist hospital place.

She's a non-urgent patient whom the ward sister had been trying to shift out of the acute ward for weeks, but couldn't because of her mental health issues.

'You've got five minutes,' Ellie had snapped. She was yelling at you because someone yelled at her, because their boss yelled at them.

'Of course, no worries,' you'd lied soothingly, with an end-of-day to-do list piling up, of patient results coming back in and urgent reviews and referrals and outpatient bookings to be done. You tapped out the medications on the chart in five minutes and gave it to her. Three other people asked you for other jobs in that time.

It turns out you had made a mistake.

You had missed out a medication. There's a page that is usually for in-hospital medication only, to avoid venous thromboembolism. For prevention of DVT in the patient population. You don't continue that medication when you leave, it's just injected every night at the hospital during a stay. You didn't spot that this patient is usually on a different, long-term anti-coagulant medication that she would continue. Her GP knows to prescribe it. It's on her repeat prescription.

But it wasn't on your list.

You fix the error and tell the pharmacy team, you thank them for noticing, and go back to your work. You don't beat yourself up. The patient was safe, and the pharmacy did their job. Errors are bound to happen when you're overworked. You had taken less than five minutes for a break across almost nine hours.

There are fewer patients to look after today. Not because they were safely discharged.

Because they died.

The patient with dementia, who rolled across the floor and refused medication and pulled out his lines. The patient who just kept bleeding, and patiently let you put that cannula in her arm for unit after unit of packed red blood cells and tranexamic acid and omeprazole. It was like filling a bucket with a hole, the organs oozing the blood, just to keep her stable for that little bit longer. Until even that didn't work.

The patient with acute kidney injury, and chronic end-stage kidney disease, whose dialysis would stop, as it was no longer helping.

It always seems to happen in the early hours. Sometime between 1 a.m. and 3 a.m.

After their last visitor has gone, and maybe they feel released. They fall asleep in lonely peace, as there is no longer anyone by their bedside, no longer a need to pretend. To feel better than they do, to sound more cheerful than they are, to have hope when they know there is none. Maybe they dream about waking up, and in that dream, decide that enough is enough. That's it. That's all they want. Sleep that is unbroken.

There's one extra body in the team, today. The reg who was due to run outpatient clinics in the next hospital turned up to discover that they'd been summarily cancelled, and was told to report to the ward. Sucks for her. She was looking forward to a week away from the stress of it, looking forward to the relative calm of sitting in clinic and helping one patient at a time. Patients who aren't going to keep deteriorating and then die on you. Patients who are well enough to walk into the consulting room and walk out again.

You take a full ten minutes for lunch. In this time, you toast your sandwich, make a coffee and go to the loo. All of this feels fairly civilised.

You do the ward jobs, and try to be helpful.

You help with a chest drain for a patient who has fluid crushing one of his lungs, and talk him down from panicking. The fluid pours down the tube and into a bottle, and after a litre, he feels the cramping pain of his lung re-expanding into its proper space. He hadn't felt much before, but now every breath hurts. He's suddenly aware of his mortality. You all are.

A respiratory consultant who has been storming around the wards, in more of a mood than usual, has gone off sick today. She'd been coughing, you'd all noticed it, but she'd refused to go home, because she didn't have a temperature. She spends a lot of her day telling people that a cough isn't enough to raise suspicion of Covid-19. But then she got a temperature after all, and everyone she coughed around is feeling uneasy, knowing that they will be next.

You start thinking about everyone in the hospital you've pissed off, says another consultant. Who'll save the last ventilator for me?

Another consultant, convinced he's been infected by a dying patient who false-tested negative, is asking if doctors can be tested privately. You think that he should be the one to know, but he doesn't.

Who knows? asks the consultant, helplessly, rushing off to another urgent referral in A&E. He says as he leaves, No one knows! No one has time to find out!

The lab test from the swab isn't that accurate. Even with the most optimistic interpretation. Some say it's as low as one in three tests giving a valid result. A lot of false negatives, from the swab not picking up enough of the virus on the sweep in the nose and down the throat. The CT imaging is more accurate, but it's not the guideline standard for diagnosis.

This means that you can't say someone has died from Covid if the computer says no on the swab test, even if the imaging and the biochemistry and the clinical signs and the contact history and the progress of the disease say it was, beyond any reasonable doubt.

If you were the suspicious type, you'd say that someone, somewhere, wanted to play down the figures.

It's hardly surprising that the respiratory consultant, who spends her time in the Blue Zone, on the Covid wards, has gone down with it. Except that she's the one with the best access to the PPE. You've had none in A&E. And when you visited the Covid patients, you wore your own clothes under the gown, because there weren't any scrubs issued for you. You left the notes and your phone outside with the nurse. The on-call consultant you were working with was visibly nervous, going into the sealed-up Covid bay, with the closed doors and aerosol-generating interventions. You'd never seen this consultant before, he's from an outpatient speciality, and you wonder if he'd been drafted unwillingly into the on-call shifts. The resp consultant looked at you crossly, for not wearing the scrubs, like it was your fault.

Only one of you needed to be in there, she barked. She was right. You should have refused to go in.

Later, the senior pharmacist comes to find you on the ward, and tells you that he's put a DATIX against you, a record of an avoidable medical error. You apologise about the medication you forgot on the patient's draft discharge notice, you explain that you were asked to do it at the end of the day under undue time pressure. That you'd have corrected it hours before the patient went on to her next hospital.

It's a learning experience, he tells you, a bit smug about the teachable moment.

He's already reported you to your consultant and your registrar. Your consultant says he wasn't even going to mention it to you, he says that maybe someone else should help you do the discharge notices, he means that as a kindness. You agree that help from someone else would be nice.

You haven't looked at your phone all day. At the end of the shift, sometime after you were meant to leave, you remember in a panic that you hadn't checked to see if your children needed you during their long home-school day, following the Google classroom directions. They didn't, they just sent a few funny emojis and requests for snacks. But you see a flurry of messages from your junior doctor cohort.

They're saying that the British Medical Association have suspended the rights to breaks and restricted hours, and fifty-six-hour weeks are not unacceptable. That weasel double negative. They're saying that the hospital administration has cancelled study days and annual leave. A colleague is saying she's been sent masks by her family in China, who are providing her with better protection than the NHS.

The respiratory ward team are saying they've run out of PPE and are expected to carry on without it. They are going to another ward and will steal their supplies, so they can get on and see and treat their Covid patients. They're saying doctors who speak out about the lack of PPE, the ones who start crowdfunding campaigns to get enough for themselves and their colleagues, are being vilified by their Trusts, and muzzled from speaking out.

Children are invincible, you repeat to yourself, again and again. You've seen the table, how the deaths rise exponentially by decade, you save it on your phone for reassurance. You're nowhere near invincible, but you'll be just about OK. The youngest death was forty-seven.

But that was a couple of weeks ago.

And this is now.

Today.

A healthy thirty-three-year-old. A young black woman. A mother of two.

She wasn't well. Short of breath.

Her family called an ambulance.

The paramedics turned up, and said there was no need to take her to the hospital.

You know yourself that's what your med reg would have said, had she turned up at Majors in a mask. What the hell is a thirty-three-year-old doing in A&E with suspected Covid? She should go home and go to bed. Drink some tea and have some paracetamol.

But they wouldn't have sent her home without checking her observations, measuring her oxygen saturations, testing her blood.

She never came into hospital.

She got worse, at home, and then she died.

She got worse. She was just thirty-three. Now it gets worse, still.

Today, you find out that a thirteen-year-old has died. Confirmed with the virus. No other health issues. Short of breath. Intubated. Ventilated. Sedated into an induced coma. Asian like you. Like your children.

And then he died. No one by his side.

Your sons are twelve and fourteen. They stand to this boy's left and right. The bodies are lining up, and the virus is picking us out, deciding who to let breathe. It's not just the old. It's not just the vulnerable. It's picking people at random, like a crazed shooter on a roof.

Any healthy young woman, young man, any healthy teenager. Anybody walking out in the open.

All at risk.

You see an email that you are no longer allowed to prescribe medications for discharge without registrar supervision. Following that DATIX.

Which is hilarious, because a registrar, with at least eight years more experience than you, would almost never do discharge paperwork and many wouldn't even know how to do it. You whine about this on WhatsApp with the junior doctors, until someone threatens to do something to help you, and you backtrack fearfully, because complaining is cathartic, but fighting the system is like picking your own scabs. Especially for something as small as this, which affects no one but yourself.

You piously retreat and say that you were glad the pharmacy team did their jobs.

You wonder how you are going to do your own job. You're going back in tomorrow and tomorrow and tomorrow. Still no scrubs, still no PPE – with the consultant who's convinced he's got it. Coughed on by the consultant who did have it. Who'll save the last ventilator for you?

Who have you pissed off, lately?

And how can you live with yourself, knowing that you are bringing this back every day, to your home? To your children.

Someone, a literary friend of yours, tweets that anyone who isn't saving lives feels pretty useless at the moment.

You feel like saying that the ones who are there with the patients, helplessly spectating on death, feel even more useless.

You're meant to be there to help. But you're just batting away an illness with your hands, palms stretched open, trying hard not to catch it yourself. You're no real help. There is no cure.

There is a woman who has been with you for weeks. You know her well. Know her extended family and her likes and dislikes. She got better and then she got worse. She is now being tested for the virus, which she must have got while in hospital. From healthcare worker or patient or patient visitor transmission.

There's not much you can do for her now.

At the end of your shift, the consultant discussed her with the palliative team, and confirmed that she was for End Of Life. EOL. It's a medical pathway for a patient expected to die in the next few days. No more active treatment. No more observations or invasive procedures. No more blood tests or ECGs. Just whatever she can manage to eat if she is hungry, whatever she wants to drink if she is thirsty. Medication for pain, for calm, for constipation. You offered to prescribe a gin and tonic, but she didn't fancy one.

Your consultant prescribes wine three times a day instead.

She's too sick to go to the hospice, and they can't take her while she is Covid positive in any case. She'll stay on the ward, in the most comfortable side room, until she passes away. There's some PPE outside her door, but not enough. Gloves, apron, gown. The most basic protection.

Nobody will go in her room, if they can help it.

You don't want to, and you thought you were one of the good guys.

That thirteen-year-old died alone. Would you ever let your child die alone, for fear of what might happen to the others?

Look after the living, they always say, the living need you more than the dead.

But we're not dead yet. She's not dead yet.

You open her door, and ask how she's doing. Ask if there's anything she needs.

She keeps her eyes closed.

Your sister kept her eyes closed, in her comfortable room in the hospice. Towards the end it was like she was already gone, and the stubborn machine of her body just kept ticking. In the calm of her final sleep, her heart was trying to compensate for her falling blood pressure, running marathons at 200 beats a minute.

And you look at your patient. Eyes closed. Asleep.

And you know it's over. But you don't want to give her up.

You just want to say, look up, wake up. Wake up.

7

Pariah

It's a sad day.

You cried when you got home.

Not for the dead. For the living. For yourself.

Your children's father is scared of you. When you come in the door, he keeps well away. He wipes the handles that you touched with ungloved hands.

He doesn't believe that you already washed your hands when you left the hospital.

He barks, You still walked through that filthy place until you got out of it. You're putting our lives at risk. A thirteen-year-old died! Didn't you know that? And despite yourself, you start to argue and justify yourself, even though you're the doctor and you know that your actions are safe and don't need defending.

There's a sink at the entrance, you tell him, and he doesn't believe you and you think that you might take a photo to prove it to him and then you think fuck it. You don't need to prove anything. And he says your clothes are dirty and you say that you wore scrubs and

he is yelling, red in the face. About your stethoscope —
which you disinfected before you hugged your kids.

They cry. You cry.

It's a sad day.

It's true. You wore scrubs. Your steth is clean. Your hands
are clean.

It's true. You spent an hour, the day before, with a patient
who is now confirmed with Covid-19. You drained
more fluid from his pleural space and peritoneum that
morning.

Once the patient's swab came back positive for Covid-
19, he was put in a side room, and started on the
Optiflow oxygen, the high-risk aerosol-producing
intervention. You needed to take the blood samples for
cross-matching so he could receive his blood transfusion.
His Hb was dropping and he was already breathless.
The nurse in full PPE in the room couldn't manage it,
he had no palpable or visible veins and you knew you
couldn't take the ultrasound in there to find a deeper
vein, as it would then be a dirty machine and couldn't
be used for other patients until it'd been properly
sterilised. Pass it over to the Cold team, said your reg,
referring to the after-hours team of doctors who cover
the wards. You knew that there was no scheduled cover
after hours for your ward that evening, as a message had
gone round the junior doctors asking if anyone could
do it. You knew that even if there was someone to take
a handover for the job, you could probably get it done
sooner, as you've spent a rotation on ITU. But you were
already an hour late.

You'd gone to the loo once in a nine-hour shift.

You ordered pizza for the children, clicking quickly through an app on your phone, and telling them to leave the box at your front door. No-contact delivery. You gathered all the equipment for the bloods. You gathered all the sterile equipment for an arterial stab, including local anaesthetic, in case that was the only way to get the samples for the blood transfusion. Disinfecting lollipops and a surgical drape.

You donned what is currently the full PPE for your Trust, which is pitiful compared to what other countries are given. The visor kept sliding down your head and gave you less protection than the sunglasses in your handbag.

The patient was apologetic about the fuss, and showed all the bruises and prick marks in his arms from previous failed attempts to take the blood.

His radial artery was obscured by a haematoma that happened earlier in the day, when you took a blood gas from the artery to confirm the oxygenation of his blood while his saturation was tumbling.

His other radial artery was obscured by a cannula dressing, which is needed for his IV antibiotics to manage his potential sepsis.

The choice was the femoral artery or the foot. The trouble with the femoral is that it can gush. And he's already anaemic. You didn't want the cure to be more damaging than the disease.

You squeezed a tourniquet around his lower limb. You put a needle in a barely there vein on his foot, and the blood was exquisitely slow in filling the bottles. You crouched to the floor to let gravity help. Your consultant was knocking on the side-room door, wondering why you were still there, in full PPE, doing procedures out of hours.

You labelled the bottles by the bedside, to be sent to the lab, instructing the nurses that an urgent transfusion would be needed that night.

You pulled off the inadequate PPE in the room, and washed your hands in the sink in the corner. As per protocol, you took off the mask and visor outside the door.

You then washed your hands. Again.

Your hair was uncovered. Your shoes were uncovered.

You forgot to put on fresh gloves to take off the mask, which you are not meant to touch with bare hands.

And when you get home, late and anxious, your children's father screams at you like you're unclean, like you're a leper, like you're the rabid dog, and not him, although his teeth are bared. You yell back, and then you cry for an hour, and then you eat the lunch that you didn't get the chance to eat on the nine-hour shift. The children come and hug you. He keeps his distance. Afraid.

How could you be so selfish? he says.

Other people say you're a hero, you're saving people's lives on the frontline, and you think of how many people would have deteriorated and died without your team, there for them, treating them. And he thinks you're selfish.

A week ago, he agreed with your outrage, when a landlady tried to evict her tenant because he worked for the NHS. She said she was sorry to throw him out without notice, but it was only a matter of time before he got ill. Stories of wronged NHS workers were flying around social media.

But you're not crying because you think you've been wronged. You're not crying at the extraordinary unfairness.

You're crying because you think he might be right.

Not all lepers have spots. Some wear scrubs in A&E. You're like Marie Curie playing with her radium. An aid worker in a camp. A bomb defuser in a war zone. A soldier against mustard gas, fumbling for a clumsy helmet. Heracles against the many-headed hydra.

A gun's a coward's weapon. An arrow is too. Shoot from a distance. Keep yourself safe. You can't be touched. You won't bleed.

But your job can't be phoned in.

You are touching the patient. Breathing the same air. Drawing their blood, tapping their fluids, and sending them off in neatly labelled bottles for blood grouping and antibody testing and cytology and culture and biochemistry.

You are talking to your patients pleasantly, about what they're going to do when they get out of this place and the world is open again.

You know you're not a hero. You're just someone doing a job. Heroes are selfish people. Vainglorious. Battle-addicts. Heroes are I, I, I. Rambo. Rimbaud.

Rimbaud said that I is someone else.

Some people are railing on social media about the insufficient PPE, the lack of equipment, the lack of support.

You know that if you didn't have it, you'd still go in to help a patient who was arresting. It wouldn't even be a choice.

You'll probably get the virus anyway. You all will. You may as well get it doing something helpful. Better to do what you're doing than hide in your home, paralysed with fear, watching your way through Netflix.

Someone else, another Muslim doctor, has died. He'd come out of retirement to help out.

It must be hard to go in, they say, day after day, your friends chatting to you on the social networks. It must be hard to go in and know you're putting yourself at risk.

The fearful face of the children's father as he backs away from you, wiping away your traces from the surfaces. The shouting, the children covering their ears, burying themselves in the downstairs duvets, diving into their screens to escape it. The tears dripping freely down your face. You haven't yet taken off your jacket. The baleful glare as you pull it off and look for a place to put it. Everything about you is unclean. Contaminated. The toxic glow surrounds you.

It's easy going in, you reply. It's coming home that is hard.

8

The Mask

It's day 11 of lockdown. The country is losing count of the dead. No longer surprised by a single loss of life. In someone young. In someone without comorbidities. The shock from two days ago is numbed by familiarity. So people are dying, they shrug, as though it's old news.

The rules are changing every day.

A week ago the consultants laughed when one of their number wore a mask to a meeting. Now you can't enter the bay in any ward without a mask, an apron and gloves.

That's changed from the day before.

A patient with liver failure who also had a cough is being kept in the side room. You take her bloods with painstaking difficulty, because she has a condition that wrecks her veins, and send them in a pod to the lab. Pathology reception call in a fury that you have sent over the blood of a possible Covid patient in a normal pod. Before it was just the Covid nasal swabs that needed double-bagging and special pods. Now it's anything to do with the patient who is suspected.

That changed from the day before.

The day before the pleural fluid from another potential Covid patient flooded over the floor of his bay, as his bottle overfilled. It was mopped up, and that was it.

Today it would be an amber-level professional clean, and the bay would be cleared while that was awaited.

The ward clerk tells you in disbelief that she isn't allowed into the non-clinical offices. The bereavement team need paperwork completing on a patient who has passed away, but they won't let her through the door, and shout out to her in the corridor. When she hands them the file, they put on gloves before they take it, treat it gingerly like contaminated waste.

You're not meant to handle files on the wards without gloves, they tell her.

That's changed from the day before.

A surgeon who needs to review a patient with a spinal injury enters your ward's doctors' office with a mask. Surgery now feels like a foreign country, where they do things differently, where the wards are hollowed out and emptied, as all elective surgeries have been stopped. He's not used to the medical wards, stuffed with patients who are suspected Covid positive. He won't talk to your team without the mask, and keeps as far from you all as he possibly can.

This is still a clinical area, he says, apologising for the mask, gesturing towards the rolling computers, the sink and the kettle in the corner. Concerned about the risk posed to him by the few minutes he is forced to spend in the same bland room where you spend much of your day.

Clinicians masking to talk to their clinician colleagues.

That's changed from the day before.

The language has changed. Instead of Blue Zone and Red Zone, the consultants say Dirty or Clean.

Is this a clean bay?

Is that a clean patient?

No, it's dirty.

No, they're dirty.

That's definitely changed from the day before.

As a coincidence, one day after the hospital got a delivery of scrubs, it has become protocol for anyone on the medical wards or A&E to wear them. Before, you were told not to wear scrubs, as there weren't enough of them, and that wearing them if you weren't directly dealing with a confirmed Covid patient was theft.

That's changed from the day before.

One of the patients isn't doing too well. He's been stepped down from ITU, where he'd been intubated. His observations, biochemistry and bloods are all improving. On paper he's as fit as you. But he's looking miserable and after his sedated stay in critical care is barely able to get out of the bed to pee.

Is anyone coming in to see you? you ask. You know that he has a wife, and kids, and local parents. No one's allowed in, the registrar whispers to you. No visitors at all now. Across the site.

You'd thought that they were allowed one visitor, at least. But that's changed, too.

Someone you respect starts saying on social media that we can't stay in lockdown just to protect 1 per cent of the population, that we'll all suffer and die as the economy suffers and sputters to a halt. He's in the vulnerable part of the 1 per cent of the population, so he's allowed to say that without sounding like a eugenicist. He's echoing what other people are saying. They're not supporting the lockdown, and they are only a few days into it.

That's changed from the day before.

There's not the backlash you expected against this anti-lockdown comment. Ten days ago, before lockdown was confirmed, there would have been retorts that they may as well decriminalise murder against the over-seventies, as the government is already getting away with it. Letting secret spreaders roam free to infect the elderly on their weekly grocery shop.

People are accepting the lack of availability of ITU beds as a practical reality, rather than a tragedy.

My brother has limited mobility and learning disabilities. He didn't make the cut.

My colleague has portal hypertension and liver cirrhosis. He didn't make the cut.

These are not people in the over-seventies bracket. They are middle-aged. They are young.

You come in the morning, and find that one of your patients, who is awaiting an organ transplant, and who was deemed not for ITU, has been made DNACPR in the night. That means Do Not Attempt Cardio Pulmonary Resuscitation. That means if her heart stops, no one will attempt to restart it. She's worked for the NHS for thirty years. People know her in the Trust.

You'd handed over to the twilight junior, just asking him to keep an eye out for her CT scan, telling him she was for full escalation, but she had been documented as preferring not to have intubation by anaesthetics. The twilight team hands over to the night team, who interpret this as a DNACPR. This is because if you come back from a cardiac or respiratory arrest, the next step of treatment would normally be intubation and ITU.

None of this was made clear to the patient. It's also critically documented in the notes by the night team that she is probably dying and that no one on the day team had told her the truth.

The night reg comes to your ward to complain about this, and has moved her to the Covid ward: exactly where the respiratory consultant had said she should not go, as it would be a death sentence for someone with her reduced immunity.

You find her in a bay full of Covid patients, with aerosol-generating oxygenation. You try to rescind the

DNACPR, showing the paperwork which shows she is due for an inpatient assessment of a liver transplant at King's. Your job is to keep her alive until then.

It just says assessment, says the consultant, not your consultant, you have just met him the day before. Doesn't mean they'll do it. They're hardly doing any transplants, now. With the situation.

But they're still calling her in, you argue.

They're cancelling appointments, they're hardly doing any, now, says the consultant. With the situation.

Like he's just learned to use this sentence, and likes the way it sounds.

The patient tests negative for the virus and you manage to get her off the Covid ward, some seventeen hours after she was taken there.

She gives you a cheerful thumbs-up, as she is wheeled out of it.

You think, this is how you die of Covid-19 without ever having the disease. Quickly, by having a cardiac arrest with suspicion of Covid, and no one will resuscitate you, as there's a DNACPR in place. Slowly, by having your assessment regarding your suitability for transplant cancelled, which means having your transplant itself cancelled, which means learning to live without a working liver, and finding out the hard way that you cannot, however much you cut down on the hard work you used to send it, quitting the booze and no longer popping pills, not even paracetamol.

You enter the side rooms and the bays looking like a villain in a children's book. Blue scrubs, cheap apron from a roll, mask and gloves. The patients look disconcerted rather than comforted by the effort. Wrapped in the scraps of plastic, you're not really wearing much more protection than a tourist in the winter. You're more protected when you walk into the hospital, because then you wear a fluffy hat and shades which protect your eyes.

The patients and some of the ward staff stop calling you by your name, as they can't really tell you apart. Anonymous warriors in blue, spilling into the hospital with regulation armour in comically flimsy protection.

You haven't seen the PPE you were trained with, which has the full hood, since the day of the training.

The patients call you She.

She's stopped my TPN.

She's taking my blood.

She's taking a venous blood gas with a syringe.

She's replacing my cannula.

I can't focus while she's doing that.

A couple of days before, your children's father was afraid of you, because he thought you weren't safe.

Today, your patients are afraid of you, because you are safe. Because you are masked and concealed. Untouchable.

They fear that they are dirty, because you are clean. That's changed since the day before.

9

Angels

It's day 12 of lockdown. Hardly any cars as you walk along the dual carriageway. The cabbages and cauliflowers are being stripped from the fields by a battered tractor, with a circular conveyor looping around it. A couple of people pass you on their bikes. No one else is walking up that road, or down it, for that matter.

The fox is still there, nestled in the weeds, and no one can witness his lonely deterioration apart from you. Sometimes a colleague passes you in their car, and you wave them on when they offer to stop. You don't know why. The fox doesn't need you as his witness. He's beyond all that.

You arrive and see a message that one of your colleagues is sick, and won't be coming in. He insists it's not Covid, just backache, and he felt it coming on all of yesterday.

That's how it starts, says another colleague, just returned from a month off, sweating out the virus alone in the hospital accommodation. Packing his feet and pillow with bags of ice cubes. Mine started with myalgia. Muscles aching all over.

The consultant on the ward isn't the one you were expecting. He's replacing the other consultant scheduled for that week, who had left late the night before, saying she was feeling rotten and was going to self-isolate. She'd been looking after a patient on another ward whom she was certain had Covid, from the travel history and the CT imaging, but the swab had been negative, so the ward hadn't been provided with the full PPE for the health workers attending to that patient.

At the beginning of the week, there had been a bay in your ward put aside just for Covid patients. Now there's a suspicious Covid patient in every bay, and in every side room. You glove up, mask up, tie apron, for every bay, for every bed.

You prepare everything outside the bay, the observations, the queries from the blood investigations, the results of the imaging, the referral conversations, you write a draft management plan, so you can have no reason to linger at the patient's bedside. Only one or two from the team go in, to limit the exposure.

But there's no protection between colleagues. The one who has just left with the virus, the one who has just come back. You share the same space, touch the same keyboards, work in a short line hopping on and off the few shared computers in the doctor's office. There's nothing you can do about that.

Almost a quarter of your colleagues are self-isolating, untested. The tests aren't freely available for staff, unless their suspicious symptoms are stopping a whole group of medical housemates from coming into work. If one person is poorly, they take a week out, but their asymptomatic housemates need to be off for two weeks.

That's more work for the rest of you, the ones who have stubbornly remained healthy, and don't live with other medics. As a reward you are given free lunches. Basic stuff, a chicken or cheese or tuna sandwich, a green apple, a packet of crisps.

There's rumour of a free chocolate egg, but you'll believe that when you see it.

You'd not managed to get so much as a compliment-ary coffee back before the cafes shut, as you just went to work and came home, and there was no time in the long day to pee let alone drink coffee. You are all quite openly pleased about the basic lunch, packed up in a brown paper bag. You all take the five minutes to go and get it.

You often think that most people are quite happy to work for food. Like authors at festivals. Or book groups.

There must be something primordial, some evolution-ary tug, that says food now beats cash later.

You sign up for the ten-pound-off voucher for the local takeaway, valid for a few days. It's a token gesture made by a big company. You're not ungrateful. You're home late every night, and you probably should have at least two meals a day to keep going. The children joke that you only eat their leftovers. It's less funny because it's true.

You manage to eat the lunch. You eat it sitting down for five minutes, in the mess, and you even toast the sandwich. You chat briefly to your colleagues about the mess mouse, who lives on the biscuit crumbs. The cleaner has given up coming to the place; it's full of infected scrubs which are dumped on the cheap sofas at the end of shift. It's not a safe place to clean.

You write out a list of ward jobs for each patient, and stay on top of the jobs. You're proud to discharge an elderly lady safely home; she's end-stage cancer, and her husband was furious that she had to stay overnight; everyone thinks a stay in hospital is a death sentence. She had to come in as her mouth is full of cancerous growth, and she can't get food past it, so she's fed straight through to her stomach. Except that the tube got displaced, and had to be replaced under X-ray guidance. She's well, the tube is in a good position, and she can start using it now it's been twenty-four hours since the procedure.

You're less proud to discharge a young man back out onto the streets, still bruised and limping from his drug-fuelled fight with a brick wall and then the pavement, all captured on CCTV, but now he's been detoxed, treated with antibiotics and declared medically fit. You organise an outpatient appointment for his probably damaged liver. No one is meant to be homeless anymore, but the hospital discharge team is sure he won't turn up to the council for his placement. He's been living in his car. He gives you the make and model like someone else might give their address.

A man with learning disabilities starts coughing, sputtering and desaturating, and it might be because he aspirated his lunch, as he insisted on self-feeding, according to the nurses. Or it might be Covid-19. He tested negative, but until then he was stuck on the Covid ward with lots of patients who were positive. The chances of a hospital-acquired infection aren't quantified, but everyone feels instinctively that they must be pretty high. You sit him up, put him on oxygen, start him on antibiotics for aspiration pneumonia while he continues to sputter, and then he vomits on you. Not so much, and mainly fluid. You carry on and look for a vein, so you can give him fluid while you keep him nil by mouth, until his swallow is tested. You order a portable X-ray to come urgently.

You ask the nursing team to swab him for Covid. Again.

Other people on the team aren't doing anything much. For once you have two more senior doctors than you need for the ward, another result of those cancelled outpatient procedures and cancelled clinics, and they have time to scroll through their emails and the news. You'd feel too guilty to do that. You don't even like sitting down. It probably annoys the other doctors, especially the senior ones, as they feel they have to stand too, when they talk to you.

And then they tell you. Scrolling through their emails. Looking at the news. A nurse is dead.

A nurse is dead from Covid-19.

A nurse in your hospital.

A nurse you know.

A nurse you worked the late shift with the other weekend.

You remember that shift. You'd been covering her ward as well as being on-call for the medical patients in A&E. You'd chatted about how you were late to medicine, and how she was late to nursing. About putting your kids before your careers. She apologised for asking you to prescribe something, and you apologised for not sorting it out before she'd had to ask you. She smiled. You smiled.

You're both so polite. You're both so similar.

She'd been off sick. Self-isolating sensibly.

And then she'd come into A&E.

And then she'd been admitted. Swabbed for Covid. And then she'd gone to ITU.

And then she'd died. Covid positive. She had two children.

She was just thirty-nine years old.

The hospital is in shock. The news spirals out in seconds to every ward to every department to every doctor and nurse. For a moment, on that afternoon, the hospital is one pulsating organism, and its lifeblood is gushing out.

Thirty-nine.

The same shift as you.

And you're here, and she's gone.

Another nurse has died, too. In another hospital. Even younger. Thirty-six.

When that young black mother died, you told yourself she'd deteriorated at home, she hadn't been in hospital, her family hadn't the information to insist she come in and be assessed, insist she be treated. You told yourself that's why such a young woman died of this disease.

But your nurse was a frontline nurse. She knew all about Covid. She had come into A&E when she could still walk. Her nursing colleague had sat with her. She'd gone to ITU. Consultants and clinicians and nurses who knew her had cared for her.

And she still died.

Dulce et Decorum est. Pro Patria Mori. The old lie.

You once thought people who went to war were stupid. Cannon fodder or toffs. Manipulated kids looking for a wage. Idiot posh kids who didn't like exams. Your ex-RAF father-in-law told you off about that. Your best friend did the same. You said you'd never let your kids fight for their country. Because that just means fighting for someone's powerful political whim, while the puppet masters sit in stately homes and drink sherry. Sleep well at night on good linen. Letting someone else take their bullets on the dirt and dry sand of the frontline.

You're not a soldier. But this is still being called the frontline. By ministers. By media. Carers for the sick taking the bullets without proper defence.

You're remembering that last shift you took with her. It was just before lockdown. Patients came in, and those who weren't suspected with Covid were put in a regular bay. Bloods were taken, and imaging was done, all without special protection. And it is only when you checked the bloods, when they came in an hour or so later, that you would see the first warning signs, typically on the white cell count, the lymphopenia. Low lymphocytes. It was only when you saw the imaging, that basic first chest X-ray, that you might see something bilateral, white shadowing on both sides of the lungs. Most infections wouldn't affect both sides of the lungs equally. No temperature yet. No spike. No cough. But you could hear it coming like distant thunder. The virus dropping heavily around you like rain in a storm.

She didn't die for her country. She died to save the dying. It wasn't her choice. She wasn't given a choice.

A Facebook post flies around with her kind smile and luminous angel wings opening around her.

Her family ask all those who knew her to light a candle for her.

The nurses post their candles on the same thread. Candles flickering in all the sad and stifling homes that spin out around the hospital.

★★★

When you need to sing happy birthday to your niece on the WhatsApp family chat, a couple of hours after you'd heard the news about your nurse, you just can't.

You'd thought for a moment you could fool them, forget her death for the time it takes to sing and make small talk while the cake is cut. But the moment you flick on the screen, you see your own face, the mouth sagging at both edges. You see everyone else in their cosy squares, cuddling children and grinning to the camera, and their smiles falter when you come on the shared screen. You've already spoiled the party. Your eyes red and swollen.

Your mother looks at your face, surprised and concerned. Like she doesn't quite recognise you.

You look tired, she says, and it's over. As she would say, the jig is up.

You hang up the call, briefly explaining why. You message quickly that if they call back, your children have the phone to sing the birthday song and chat.

The kids don't do a great job with the small talk; they throw your phone around to each other like a hot grenade. They have no sense of polite diplomacy. Not yet.

You feel bad for your niece. Your sister's daughter. Her birthday song. It should have been all about her. You should have faked the smile, faked the song. Worn the mask. If someone asked you how you were, you should have just said, Fine, like everyone expects.

Don't burden people with the truth. Not your truth, at least, it's not their problem.

People want happiness and humour.

Nothing's funny if it's true.

You sit alone in the kitchen, scrolling obsessively through the tributes to the nurse, who was much like you. Your friend messages you, panicked, as she has seen the news. Knows that's your hospital.

That was your shift. It could have been your disease. It could have been your death.

Don't see patients, your friend says, if you don't have proper gear.

The proper gear is laughable.

No one's refusing, as if you refuse to see a patient, refuse to investigate a patient, refuse to manage a patient, they will die.

People will die anyway, she says.

Not in front of you, you reply flatly. Not when you know you can stop it.

You're not a soldier, she says.

You're not. Soldiers are helpless. They watch, while comrades die.

Dulce et Decorum est.

An ecstasy of fumbling. Fitting the clumsy helmets just in time.

But someone still is drowning.

In all my dreams, in all my sleepless nights – I see her before me, drowning.

Don't go in, she says. Say you're sick. Lie. Just lie. Say the kids are sick.

You wanted to help, all your life. To make a difference. And now you've been given what you always wanted.

The chance to help.

You're not a liar. You're a storyteller. There's a difference.

Colleagues have been taking time off for the sniffles, joining their partners who are on leave.

Colleagues have suddenly been claiming chronic backache.

They're not going to say they have Covid. As when they come back, they'd be told they could be put in the highest-risk wards, as they're most likely to be immune.

So, you're not a soldier. And neither was the nurse who died. Or the other nurse. Or the other doctors. You could die, just the same.

But you're not a liar, either. You can't lie to save yourself.

You see the tribute from the hospital. The angel meme. You forward it on social media.

'We are heartbroken. We will forever remember her...' Her smile. Her kindness. Her care.

People are always calling nurses the angels of the NHS. It's a hard title to live up to. Like they don't have the right to complain or bitch in huddles like anyone else.

You tell your friend, if anything happens to me, look out for my kids. And don't let *them* speak at my funeral. Don't let *him*, either. Seriously.

Your friend laughs. She doesn't ask why. She knows why.

You're no angel, either.

10

Soldiers

It is day 13 of lockdown. It's April now.

April Fool's Day came and went without anyone on the junior doctors' feed being able to work out what was a joke or not. Someone posted a fake document stating that everyone would have to stay in their same rotations, in their same hospitals all year, without the planned move in August, without continuance of training, without annual leave, and nobody was surprised. It's not funny if it might be true.

Confirmed UK cases: 38,168

New cases: 4,450

UK deaths: 3,605

You're tired (yes, you're always tired) and so you write this bullet point fast, after the children are in bed, after you have dutifully responded to friends and family, squinting with only one eye open at a time so you can rest the other one, lying on your belly on the floor, fingers pattering like rain over your slow little laptop.

The echo chamber of social media is humming about the deaths of doctors and nurses. Another nurse, young and unprotected. A midwife.

Elderly doctors are coming out of retirement, foolishly fearless, to work in unfamiliar environments with new and untested rules.

Henry Marsh, recently retired neurosurgeon, goes on record in the *Financial Times* to say he will come back if he is asked. Despite falling in the high-risk group since his recent birthday, a modest gathering which he thinks transmitted Covid-19 to his vulnerable wife.

Others say that doctors and nurses should stop bleating, that no one forced them into their jobs, that they knew what they were getting into. That if they didn't want to get sick, they shouldn't have trained in healthcare.

The stinging unfairness of this casual accusation should be obvious, but it isn't shot down. Instead it is retweeted enough times to give it equally unfair volume.

The rules changed. No one knew what we were getting into.

No one trained in medicine thinking they were going to be put in danger.

No one flew to the UK from their home country thinking they were going to give their lives to the NHS.

You trained with the graduate-entry medics. You trained with a dancer, who was debating between engineering and medicine as he hit his late thirties, and you can't remember why medicine won out. You trained with a musician, who headlined well-known indie festivals. You trained with a mum who was a lawyer, and who thought she had better get a kinder job, with her suited partner out of the picture and a family to care for. You trained with former nurses, who had got frustrated with the doctors they worked with, thought they could do a better job, and went for the medical degree to prove it. You trained with an Oxbridge rich kid, a talented choral singer whose family were all doctors, and who had never thought there was anything else she could do. You trained with a lab scientist, a pharmacist, a physics lecturer, a classics schoolteacher, a psychologist, an epidemiologist, an accountant, a banker, an Olympic athlete.

And in your third year, you were mixed with those who were doing medicine as their first degree. Parents in medicine or parents with ambition, teenagers who played the game, with ambition, too. On their induction day, they said, Whoop-whoop! We're gonna be DOCTORS!

Everyone cheered, unembarrassed by their vaulting ambition.

There's a scene in *Blackadder Goes Forth*, when the soldiers talk about signing up for the army, the act which got them in the trenches, for the Big Fight against Fritz and the Krauts.

The girl who kissed Baldrick is described wryly as the first casualty of the war.

The Nice-But-Dim private talks about leapfrogging down to the office with his college gang to enlist.

Blackadder says how he never expected to see action or any weapon more pointed than a sharpened mango.

No one imagined anything as horrible as this war, he says.

And then they go over the top. The frontline. Cannon fodder. While the general eats at a laid table with a cloth in a stately home.

In the last frame, the poppies bloom like blood on the broken ground. Birdsong increasing in volume.

The birds have got louder now, heard with insistent clarity as the traffic is silenced. No one expected this. You're not in the army, you're not a policeman in an acronym-filled TV production. You never expected to risk your life in the line of duty.

But suddenly everyone talks as though you are.

You feel at an oblique angle to the rest of the world, sitting in their apartments in their underpants, watching TV and raking through the online news and networks. Doom-scrolling on social media. Calling out to be heard in their solitude. Peevish, plaintive, playful, their hostage videos broadcast from their cells. Singing, and dancing, and baking sourdough and banana bread.

You go to work, and return. You see colleagues, drifting in shifts, and speak to them. You rarely see the same person twice in a week as you are all scattered between the twilights, the nights, the weekends and the sick-leave cover. There is no effective social distance in the hospital apart from in the non-clinical areas. You can't help a senior stabilise a patient with two metres between you. The admin staff in the non-clinical offices are meticulous about sticking out a ten-foot pole and not even touching you with that.

The weekend is different. When you're not working the weekend, you do what you would normally do. Exercise, watch TV, make pancakes for the children, play with them in the garden or kitchen. Take pathologically long baths, sometimes joined by the children, who hop in to play with their novelty plastic ducks while you scroll through your emails. Albert Quackstein with glasses and Duck Vader all in black are the favourites. Sometime you get the names wrong, and call them Albert Duckstein and Darth Duck instead, and they point out the mistake like it really matters.

You usually pick up your groceries from the garage at the end of the road. The rest is delivered online, if you get a slot, or collected from the farm shop or the fishmonger.

But this weekend, almost two weeks into lockdown, you've run out of pharmacy stuff. The unscented lotion for the eczema-prone skin. Toothpaste. Antihistamines for worsening hay fever.

You walk into town for the first time in weeks. There are people on the streets, walking with their children or family members, swerving to avoid you. Pressing themselves into the wall, and appreciative when you step out into the nearly empty roads instead. All the cafes are shut. All the restaurants. All the businesses.

You knew it had happened. You just hadn't seen it for yourself.

The pharmacy, when you get there, is shut. It has reduced opening hours now.

The supermarket opposite has a stretched line outside it, with customers waiting on the tape markers. You find the toothpaste and Piriton there.

No lotion. You suppose that the children will have to make do with the tub of gloopy ointment you have at home, combined with the various mini-lotions from the holiday travel sets.

You buy the children their favourite yoghurt to have with breakfast. There's no flour left on the shelves for baking, so you buy them cookies too.

You feel guilty and uncomfortable, just being outside with no great purpose. You feel judged. You have no inclination to walk the extra minute to the seafront, to stop and take in the view. You have no urge to stroll through the park on the way home, a detour of another few minutes. You walk home hurriedly. Couples in masks give you a wide berth. When you say thank you to those who allow you to pass, they look at you sharply. As thought you are no longer allowed to acknowledge each other anymore. As though words could cause transmission.

Some idiots vandalised the 5G masts for exactly this reason. Covidiots is trending.

Sideways look. Wide berth. People drawing back into their doorways, cowering against the walls as you pass.

You feel fugitive. You feel feared.

It is a vast relief to open your front door. To play swingball in the small sanctuary of your back garden.

You video call your family. You WhatsApp your friends. You rejoin their lives briefly, as simply as dropping downstairs to the little kitchen gatherings that have been taking place all this time, before retiring to your own life apologetically, gratefully.

You do not tell them how you are, when they ask you. You feel a little pestered as they expect you to complain, to dish the dirt. You do not wish to monopolise the conversation.

You don't want to talk at all, really. You're too afraid that you'll lose it, crumple with tears or anger, when they ask you how you are.

Medics don't ask how you are. They already know how you are. How it is.

When you're not at the hospital, you all turn displacement activity into an art form. Circulating offers and memes, setting up online quizzes.

You put the children to bed, finish the prosecco you inexpertly opened for the Zoom dinner party, and fall asleep twice at your keyboard.

You have a noisy, busy family. But loneliness is tiring, too.

People have been buying freezers. More have been bought in a week than are usually bought in a year. They are clearing the freezer aisles.

You think they'd do better with tins that you can open with a ring pull, or a Swiss Army knife. You don't know when and if the electricity will stop running. The family is filling old milk bottles with water, and storing them in the kitchen. You imagined you'd be in your crumbling house in France when Armageddon kicked off, an old ruin with land and a well, and free fuel in the surrounding forest for the wood burner. You'd live off the fruit and veg, and keep chickens, and draw water from the well, and fish in the river.

The flaw in this plan. You can't travel to second homes, unless you're a TV chef ready to be vilified by social media. You didn't think that you'd never be able to get there.

The person you most want to talk to about all of this is the one who is no longer here. That's the case with any bereavement, you suppose. That's common to all guilt.

It doesn't make it easier, just because it happens a lot.

What's happened in the world has demonstrated that with conviction.

You know, you tell your sister, speaking to the dried-out flowers and her cards littering the corner of your kitchen table, *you* didn't imagine anything as horrible as this.

She bristles. She hated being described as without imagination, though she would frequently say that she wasn't creative, with a casual shrug like she didn't care, that it was an irrelevance. You remember that she used to draw at school, she drew girls diving into deep water with bold, impetuous strokes. She sketched so well and you can't remember why she stopped.

But then she shrugs, in unusual agreement with you. Well, she says, who did?

Someone did. Scientists had been talking about a Virus X for years. How it would travel on planes and trains and cars, and slink across surfaces, and sink under our skin. But most people didn't pay attention.

A few months ago, twelve weeks ago exactly, her biggest fear was her child ploughing A levels, her child missing out on an Oxbridge first, all because of her too-early death. She felt guilty about that, you knew, and it was somehow worse that she was utterly blameless, so she couldn't even say sorry to them to make herself feel better.

Now there are no A levels. No grades at university. Medics are being graduated as practising doctors without even sitting finals.

Her children are spending what was meant to be exam season on sunloungers. If that were you, you'd be refreshing your phone screen every few moments with a FOMO bordering on obsessive, because there is so little else to obsess about.

Some people are using lockdown as some kind of self-caring opportunity. They are eating for entertainment, posting their successes and comical failures on Insta. They are bloody-mindedly exercising more than they ever did, now that they've been told they're only allowed a single out-of-doors hour. They are drinking from midday to chase away the time as urgently as boredom. Lockdown etiquette: You get to be a chunk, a hunk, a drunk.

I don't know how you can go to work, she says. Picking at you like a wasp. It's selfish. It's unsafe. I don't know how you can put your children through it.

You said exactly that about driving them around in a second-hand VW people carrier, you point out.

I stand by that, she snaps. And for the record, I don't think you're a hero. I don't think you're brave. I think you're just a mildly talented eccentric who's stumbled into a stupid time to start medicine.

You're right, you say. Thank you.

Sometimes, even though the light was never flattering, you felt that she was the only one who saw you.

11

Frontline

You've stopped looking at the news, it only depresses you. The death toll. More deaths today than yesterday. You figure that if there's something you really need to know, someone will email you.

You've stopped looking at your nhs.net emails; there are dozens of them, all usefully with the same Covid-based generic heading.

Covid-19. Covid. Covid news. Covid changes. COVID. COVID-19. Covid update. Covid situation. Covid. Covid-19.

You figure that if there's something you really need to know, someone will tell you.

You've stopped listening to what people want to tell you.

You don't attend to the messages on your phone.

You walk out of the mess when you hear them talking about the twenty-three-year-old nurse who died, the midwife who died. The constant battering of bad news isn't allowing the old bruises to heal.

The other old news they're bickering about is that all holiday is cancelled, at least until July. They've also cleared and restarted all the rotas from scratch. You make an activity out of rewriting your rota in bright pens, with the hours you're working against each day, so the children will know when you'll get home. You're now working on your son's birthday.

One of the junior doctors, a senior house officer, says she is now expected to work a full week, and then cover a weekend of on-call twelve-hour shifts, and then be back at work on Monday. No protected zero day.

I didn't want to come in today, she says. I wanted to resign.

Everyone is feeling powerless and humiliated by the more powerful bodies in the hospital, in the management offices, for daring to ask for their time off.

The rota coordinators and management staff are all taking their holiday as normal.

They don't care about us, says another junior doctor. That's why so many of us are dying. We're just expendable bodies in scrubs. *They* wouldn't work like this.

Who are *they*? Everyone who can keep their distance. Everyone who made the decision that ended up leaving doctors with inadequate protection. That a jolly, plucky British, take-*that* to the virus will make up for the fact that you are fighting an insidious illness with a plastic apron and a paper mask.

The prime minister is in hospital, someone WhatsApps the group. This is the sort of thing that breaks through the noise. But you don't really care, one way or another. You would have, before, felt something. Triumphant that his policy decisions have turned around and bitten him on the arse. The UK brought to you by Netflix, final season plot twist. You feel frustrated that he has managed to martyr himself.

Fearful that if it can happen to him, it can happen to anyone.

But you're too tired to join the twittering masses and manufacture any opinions at all. You go to bed tired and you wake up tired.

You make breakfast for your kids. Pancakes. Cereal. Yoghurt. Sliced fruit. Milk.

You hug them goodbye and pull on your cheapest clothes at the door. Clothes that you don't like, and if you have to burn or boil them, you'll cope.

You stuff the clean scrubs that you stole the night before in your handbag. They are mismatched, but you don't mind. There aren't enough scrubs to go around in the mornings, when you get in. So now you do what the theatre staff usually do, and put a set aside the night before as soon as a new batch comes in from the laundry.

You walk to work along an empty road, in the sunshine.

One of the fields has been stripped of the brassicas, and is tilled and brown. Your hay fever is still pretty bad.

You sneeze when you pass the weedy patch enveloping the dead fox, like a cautionary tale or an Aesop's fable.

You excuse yourself automatically, even though there is no one to hear you.

You go in the door, past the new mothers in pyjamas who are smoking illegally outside, and get changed.

On the ward, you go through the patients' observations, and see that one is spiking a temperature. A new patient on antibiotics. You look at the blood results. Low lymphocytes.

You order an urgent chest X-ray, a portable one which is done on the ward with the patient still in bed, and compare it with the one taken three days before. The patchy consolidation is rising up the lungs, from the base to the midzone. Antibiotics should have helped. One reason why they're not helping, is if it's viral.

You isolate the patient, ask a nurse to swab her, and put her in a side room. Her son calls and you tell him, with her permission, that she is being swabbed for Covid, that her chest X-ray is worse. You tell the truth, when you would all prefer if you could have said something reassuring, instead.

It's just a precaution. Just another test we need to run. Just a thing we have to do for everyone.

On the ward, you find out that the patient who aspirated and coughed and sputtered and threw up on you on Friday, confirmed Covid negative, was re-swabbed, and still Covid negative. Then re-swabbed again. Confirmed positive.

Third time's the charm.

It's only a matter of time before you get it. Having fluids thrown up from the throat and coughed out from the lungs is the highest-risk contact you can have. It's usually eight or nine days. It can be up to three weeks.

You find it oddly comforting to think that you will be symptomatic in eight or nine days. At least you know. Everyone else is falling like flies.

You go the mortuary, as you have been asked to identify the lady you looked after two weeks before, before she moved wards. She's been in the fridge for almost ten days. She doesn't look like she is sleeping. She looks like she's dead. She's cold, of course. Her body has hardened, and as you palpate for devices under the skin, it's like tapping a rock. You pull off your mortuary-issued apron, which is stiff and yellow, pull off the gloves, the mask. You don't know why you have to wear the mask, she's got no breath in her, no air could be squeezed from those stiff lungs. And you can't infect her, she's beyond that now.

When your sister came out of the fridge door, she looked like she was sleeping. Her cheeks were soft when you kissed them.

You had used your mother's scarf to bind her jaw shut, before they took her down to the cold storage. She was to be seen by female friends and family after you washed and wrapped her body with gloved hands, the sleeves of your dark suit rolled up. Her suit, actually. She'd given it to you years ago, for a work thing, and you'd never given it back. You'd forgotten about the stolen suit, but you bet she hadn't. You imagine her clocking you and banking the intel to use on you later; she'd have loved that.

Hot, soapy water poured under your sister's sheet, you counted as you wiped her body, and the kind volunteers shook their heads and said, So Young, So Young. Her mouth remained closed, after the binding was unwound. You all used to laugh about the family slack jaw, the soup dribbling from the lips of elderly uncles and aunts. You were cruel about them, in the casual way that children are cruel. She'd have been horrified to think she could ever be mistaken for one of the slack-jawed relatives. You're relieved the scarf worked.

You had to resist the urge to tidy her eyebrows in front of the volunteers from the mosque, who had been guiding you with such care and firmness. They saw your vanity for her anyway. No make-up, they said to you warningly. They gave you varnish remover to take off her scarlet manicure which her daughter had done for her in the hospice. They gently covered her hair in death with part of the sheet she was wrapped in, and fussed over the short curls which strayed out, as short hair couldn't be put back as neatly as long hair, in the three traditional plaits. She had never covered her hair in life, although she had sometimes covered her lack of hair during chemo. You remember that photo of her, beautiful and bald.

Is that everything, asks the friendly girl in the mortuary. You don't know how she remains so relentlessly cheerful in this job, in this cold basement, with these shelves lined with boxed cadavers. You don't ask her how she does it, or why. She levers the trolley up high, so the body can slide back into its place.

Yes, thanks so much, you say. That's everything. Thank you for your help.

That's all right, she says, surprised by your gratitude. It's my job.

You go back to your ward. You drain fluid from an abdomen, under the supervision of your reg. You'd like to do it with ultrasound, but it's not available, one machine is broken, the other is needed in day surgery. You can't borrow the ITU machine anymore, because it sits in a Blue Zone, a dirty zone, and it's not safe to bring on the ward. You don't need the ultrasound, the abdomen is so distended with fluid that it leaks out before you've finished administering the anaesthetic with a short needle. You draw back when the anaesthetic is given, and the syringe fills with the clear ascitic fluid. There's no risk of piercing the bowel in that shallow space.

You fill the bottles with the ascitic fluid for testing. Cytology, biochemistry, protein. You check the tracing of a heart. You manage soaring blood sugars. You call the hospice. You chase the referrals. You prescribe the controlled drugs. You brief the nurses on the protocol for a surgical procedure in the morning. Nil by mouth six hours before. Early breakfast if the patient wants it. Take the bloods to test the clotting by 7.30 a.m., so you can check the results at 8.30 a.m. and correct it with Vitamin K. And take another set if it's not corrected, and order fresh frozen plasma for the procedure. Two bags before the procedure. One bag during. One bag after. You give them the printed blood forms.

You walk home.

You admire the children's work.

They start fighting about something stupid, the death of a virtual llama, the malicious uncharging of a tablet, the design on a painted pot, an insult at the table, and you shout at them, and then you start crying. And then the ones who started it start crying, too.

You all say sorry. You all hug.

Sorry about your llama. Sorry about your tablet. Sorry for what we said about the pot. Sorry for the insult at the table. You're not a jerkface. You're not a noob. You're not a boomer.

And you run them a bath.

Are you still there? You're not sure. You're falling asleep writing this.

You're going to bed tired and you're going to wake up tired. You're always tired. You should worry that you're not safe to work, but it's the other way around. Work isn't safe for you.

Two more bits of news filter through, from your ignored emails and ignored WhatsApp feeds.

You're being shifted to the Intensive Care Unit that week. You find out on a group email, with lots of names you do not recognise, with the casual notice, As you are aware, you'll all be reallocated to ITU.

You weren't aware. No one asked you. No one told you. Your ward team definitely don't know.

And now the prime minister is in Intensive Care, too. That must mean intubation, ventilation, sedation, you think. That must mean weeks on a machine and a significant chance of never coming off it.

You're too tired to care, either way.

You're living in a place where even the prime minister and the future king aren't spared the bullet. The difference is that no one will let them die of it. No one will let them go gently into the night, the way that all the ordinary people have. The blond muppet's illness will be headline news, it is headline news already, and everyone will be distracted by the live-tweeted progress of this mendacious middle-aged man, burying the rest of the dead and the dying silently. Buried like bad news.

You can all catch it.

But you're not all in it together.

12

Fighter

It's day 15 of lockdown.

You're a few minutes late for work this morning, with the children bickering, and this would usually cause you to panic, but you feel that careless ennui from lack of sleep.

Are they going to fire you? asks your son, hopefully.

They aren't going to fire you. If they did, it might be a relief. You'd be let off the hook.

It's such a nice day you don't need to wear your jacket. It seems ridiculous that only a week ago you were wearing that jacket, with fluffy boots, woolly gloves and a bobble hat. You were probably wearing it all for protection rather than warmth. Trying to shield yourself from the world in a way you can't do at work, with gloves and a plastic apron. Your mother-in-law calls them plastic pinnies with obvious disapproval at how laughable they are as protection, they'd just about protect you from a soup spill, they'd do nothing about a virus sprayed into your environment.

The birds are singing, careless too. Almost reckless, they wing and spin about close to you, they are teeming in the branches and loud and proud, with almost no traffic and just the odd pedestrian, like yourself, wandering into their territory like a tourist at a heritage site. It's their world, now. You acknowledge that, acknowledge them, and carry on.

The children have been playing up, and you feel helpless to stop them fighting among themselves. They go stir-crazy at home when you take a stand and switch off their games and TV, so they can pick up the laundry festering on their bedroom floors. They throw furniture about, insult each other, and you feel bad for them, and they feel bad for you.

Last night, you all ended up camping in the living room, on a mattress on the floor, with a duvet, pillows and sleeping bags strewn on the sofas, so you can at least spend the night together if you can't spend the day.

You don't know when you will be able to spend another day off with them. It's the Easter holidays, but all your holiday has been scrubbed off with the change in rota, and won't be honoured. You can't rebook it, as no new leave is allowed for the next two months.

The newsfeeds and WhatsApp groups are buzzing about the prime minister. The news of the rising death toll of the NHS staff, the doctors and nurses and others, is buried and muffled and muted. When your nursing colleague died, she was the sixth. Now there are more than thirty.

There are officially 6,000 deaths in hospitals of Covid-19 patients. People say it's more like 7,000. You think it's

FIGHTER

so much more, as you know that many people have died
of Covid without being diagnosed on the lab test. And
so they hesitate to put it on the death certificate. You
see this in passing in the bereavement office, coming
across the paperwork of a patient who was confirmed
radiologically with Covid, but whose death certificate
says it was because of his chronic ulcerative bowel
condition. It's blatantly wrong, he died of a horrible
infection in his lungs. But no one is going to unwrite
what has been written. You know of one very senior
doctor who recommended writing Covid as a diagnosis
for another patient, even though the lab test said no; he
was berated and called back to the bereavement office,
to correct his notes.

And the prime minister, in ITU, he is getting more
attention than the thirty dead caregivers, than the 7,000
plus hospital deaths. Seven thousand. It's a number just
large enough to visualise, an Ariana Grande concert.
You can look around and see them from your festival
stage. The swelling ranks of the dead. Furious and fists
shaking, that they were taken needlessly and too soon.
Avoidable deaths.

It turns out that the PM is not even on invasive
ventilation, and you wonder why they would waste an
ITU bed for someone just on oxygen, which could
be managed on any and every ward. In ITU there is a
nurse beside the bed, day and night, in case of sudden
deterioration. Taking observations several times an
hour. If they need to pee, or get medication out of
the fridge a few steps from the bedside, someone else
takes their place. You wonder if there's more to the

story, like Churchill's concealed heart attack during the Second World War. You suspect that the news is being judiciously managed, that the public are being managed like a fractious child.

'He'll get through. He's a fighter,' says the second in command stupidly, as though the 7,000 dead weren't fighters themselves, but weak and complicit. As though they had a choice.

You don't blame this government spokesperson for being stupid. He has no constitutional right to govern, as far as you can tell, he has simply been appointed from the cabinet of career politicians as the one least likely to fuck up while the prime minister is unnecessarily taking up an ITU bed for oxygen and fifteen-minute observations. You wonder if he's been proned, at least, there's good evidence for that position helping the lungs. One ITU consultant winsomely calls it Tummy Time, as though the two nurses and doctors on each side, and the anaesthetist at the head of bed, are simply rolling over a child. And it is odd, for a moment, to think of the PM made childlike and prone by the NHS, put on his knees by the doctors and nurses he has not helped.

On the ward, a patient has died in the early hours. It is always in the early hours, you know you've said that. She needs certifying. Another patient is hypercalcaemic and dangerously anaemic. Another is spiking a temperature and shifted to a side room.

Death and deterioration have been impossibly normalised.

You're living in impossible times.

The day is busy and flies past quickly. You find out that the nurse who was with you when that aspirating patient vomited has taken the week off to self-isolate. She refuses to have her temperature taken: it's possible she was afraid that her symptoms would be dismissed. She has lost people to Covid, and she is terrified that she might have it, that she might have passed it on.

Your consultant has mentioned on the ward round that his wife is self-isolating, she is another doctor in the same hospital, but you didn't really pay attention to that while you were examining the patients, scribbling notes and charting medications. But when you go back to the doctor's office, you see that your consultant is now wearing a mask, and keeping himself apart in the corner. He says only nice things about you to the surgery team, whom you have bleeped. And then he tells you what has happened. It turns out that the consultant's wife is confirmed Covid positive, as of a few minutes ago, so he has to return to his home to self-isolate with her. He is remaining, with his mask, for a few moments, simply to organise cover for his post as he leaves.

You leave on time today. There are two more doctors allocated to the ward, so the work is spread out more reasonably. As you walk home, you're thinking about the deteriorating patients, the investigations you've requested which might not happen until the next day. The suffering on the patients' faces that swim before you.

And you're thinking about the car ride that you shared with your consultant, who offered you a lift just the other day, who has been living with a Covid-positive partner without realising it.

You check messages and see outrage. Easter bank holidays have been cancelled with no notice, just a prosaic message on WhatsApp.

You check your email and see another about your move to ITU. You'll be going along with the surgical teams who have no intensivist experience.

These are impossible times.

You know it was always impossible for someone, somewhere in the world; that some people have always lived with this stifling fear of contagious disease and death, in refugee camps, in shanty towns, in villages, but now that there are enough white middle-class people affected, it counts enough to be reported.

You get home to find out that someone has organised a clap for Boris.

You are at a loss to understand why.

No one in your street does the NHS clap, anyway. Just your immediate neighbours. You hope they don't do it just because of you.

You don't wish the prime minister any harm, you certainly don't wish him dead, but as everyone says, you are unsure the feeling is mutual.

You post about the patient who vomited on you while you had no PPE beyond the plastic pinny. Your mother-in-law's quaint phrasing. You write the emotive lines impetuously and unapologetically.

You're keeping your promise to protect your patients. You are unable to keep the promise to protect yourselves.

Everyone is afraid, and you're surprised you're not, anymore.

You're not even afraid for your children. They understand, now, that death is something that happens to mothers, and that everything just carries on. They saw that with your sister, and they have learned, too soon, that they will one day see it with you.

When you tell them you don't want a particular person speaking at your funeral, they casually ask if you want to write a list. You give them a list. You don't want him. You don't want her, either. You've given them enough time and effort in your life, and you resent the kindness you've shown. You don't want to give them the chance to monopolise your death, too.

Why would they clap for the PM? Being sick, being terminally sick even, doesn't make you a good person.

It doesn't make you right.

You imagine your sister snapping to attention at this slight. Head jerked up, meerkat alert.

You don't quite mean it. It's not that the dead aren't good. It is simply that you must be good for the dead. For the dying.

You're not allowed to insult them.

But you don't have to applaud them, either.

13

Coward

It's day 16 of lockdown, and you wake up tired, again, and see that over a thousand people have retweeted your message, and are asking where you're based, and why there's no PPE. Someone sees that they've written a whole article about you abroad, and emails it to your NHS email, under the headline 'International Doctor Has NO PPE'. Someone on social media snidely points out that you had PPE before, so where's it gone? You don't bother to explain that the PPE is for the Covid-positive patients or those with high enough suspicion for testing. You now don't use it until someone's symptomatic, and they can be infectious long before that. Someone else takes a screenshot of your Twitter bio, pointing out that you're a writer of fiction. Someone else uses it to wish the PM ill, which is a bit tasteless given that he is already in ITU. The nurses there have enough to be dealing with, without a figurehead dying on their watch.

And that's where you'll be going. Weeks ago, when the note went out asking which juniors had ITU experience, you had dutifully replied. It didn't occur to you to ignore it, although you then got a surprisingly grateful response, which made you think that other people had.

Yesterday you were on the recipients list for a group email, which said, Pending your move to ITU this week.

No one has said anything to you in person about it, but that's not that unusual, in the current situation. But your supervising consultant doesn't know about you being moved off her ward team, which is unusual.

You thought it was probably a mistake. You thought it was probably a note for the surgical juniors, who have so little to do, with elective operations cancelled, they are being sent home after the ward round at midday.

But then there was another note, more pointed, saying to turn up for ITU training, with a place and a time and an attendance list. Definitely not a mistake. This is news to your current consultant of the week, when you ask for the time off to go to the compulsory session. He says he's probably out of the loop, as he is filling in for the other consultant whose wife is Covid positive, who was himself filling in for the consultant who is self-isolating after treating a Covid-positive patient.

You don't know what it's like on ITU since you moved off the rotation, but you have heard that the older consultants are ill or self-isolating. That the doctors need to do long hours in full PPE on the unit. That everyone does twelve-hour shifts to avoid cross-contamination of staff.

You suppose that the next time a Covid-positive patient throws up on you, you'll at least be fully gowned up with a visor. You're a little afraid, because part of you wants to work there, in the place of most exposure, because it's where you think you'll help the most. You're trained to put in a central line, straight through to the heart, if someone is supervising. You can put in an arterial line by yourself. You can manage an airway, until an airway-trained anaesthetist or intensivist turns up with the evil-looking instrument to intubate. It looks like something from medieval torture, impossibly hard and pointed, so alien to the soft flesh of the tongue and the tender epiglottis and the vocal cords it divides down in the trachea.

You're afraid that a little bit of you wants to be in the place of highest risk. You wonder what this says about you.

You wrote a whole book criticising your father for being a gambler. And although you can shuffle and cut a deck like a pro, you never thought you were much of a gambler yourself. Strangers on Twitter are telling you to quit your job, because you've got four children. Like you're indulging in a reckless leisure activity, just by being a doctor.

Skydiving. Rock climbing. Bungee jumping.

These never appealed to you, so why does this? Maybe you like being humourless and pious about helping people.

Maybe you have an unhealthy pride in risking your life for others.

That old lie. Dulce et decorum est.

There's something distasteful about it, as blatant as a zealot knight on another selfish crusade, leaving a family behind to fend for themselves.

One of your colleagues is messaging you privately, desperate to get out of the ITU switch, he is sure that you must feel the same way. You demur, saying that you'd rather stay on your medical ward, of course you would, but you can't see a way out of it, if you're needed. He's not happy about the redeployment, and already writing to the administrators, making a case, so he can stay on the acute medical take.

If this is your last day on a medicine ward, it's actually a good day.

The sun is shining. No jacket required. The streets are eerily empty and the birds fill the silence gleefully. You don't even have to look for cars when you cross the road to the shady side.

You have clean scrubs with you, picked up the night before, to change into when you walk in the door. You've found a bathroom ten seconds from the maternity entrance, where you change. You spend less than two breaths in the building in your home clothes. You open the doors with your elbow, and twist shut the lock with a tissue to avoid touching the handle.

Only two people die that day on your ward.

One in the morning. Peacefully in his sleep.

Another practically mid-conversation with someone else in her bay. First she was there, chatting away, and then she wasn't. It took a few moments for the person beside her to realise she wasn't joking, doing a bit. The nurses think it's a good death, as far as they go. She was comfortable and in good spirits until the end.

Someone else is dying, and barely aware of her environment. She's deteriorated since coming in the night before. She doesn't ask for someone to come in with their phone or iPad, so she can chat to her relatives and say goodbye, although you do it anyway. She's just drowsy, non-rousable, and sleeping until the end. She barely acknowledges her son on the phone, on the screen. You put your hand on her arm, and hope that she will think it's her son's hand, when she hears his voice on the line, behind her shuttered eyes and shutting down consciousness. That little lie is all you have to give her, apart from the medications you are writing up for comfort. Morphine, and the anti-sickness medication that has to come with it for the opiate-induced nausea. Something for secretions from the lung, something for discomfort from the sluggish bowel.

You don't know if these patients had Covid, but they didn't die from it. They died from their long-term condition. Covid stole their relatives from their sides, the hand to hold theirs.

One man is discovered on the ward round to have signs, and the usual panic happens, as he is swabbed and moved to a side room, and everyone involved in his care starts to check their temperature obsessively.

The doctor's room is empty by 2 p.m., and you realise that you're the only sucker not having a lunch break, so take yourself off to find your free sandwich and toast it in the mess. You suppose that if coronavirus doesn't get you, the turned chicken mayo will instead. You're fairly sure it's been sitting in the crate in the canteen since 11 a.m., but you eat it anyway. You check your phone and see a few hundred messages from the doctors' WhatsApp groups, all about the cancelled leave.

You had already sent a note explaining why you couldn't work the bank holiday, should they request this formally. They won't reply to you.

What are they gonna do? says a colleague. Fire you?

He reminds you of the tweet you wrote that accidentally went viral, and you check your Wikipedia, and get your colleague to take off all the over-personal details that an ITU doctor had put on for a joke, as he was sure that no one would be looking at it. Some details of your hospital placement were there, and you don't want to risk patient confidentiality being compromised.

You finish on time. You think about the nine hundred who died that day in the country.

You think about the others who will die, because there are no other services.

You think about the dermatologist and the other specialist consultants, who are picking up a steth for the first time in fifteen years, to go on the acute medical take. You finally see the point of having to do eight years' general training before you specialise. Just in case there's a pandemic.

No one ever thought it would happen until it did.

You think about those grieving for their lost loves and lives, unsure of what will happen next.

You're all unsure.

Jobs that are lost might not be plucked up from the ground where they were abandoned.

People complain about minutiae that have suddenly grown like space-occupying brain lesions, pushing out all sense of everything else: that unpaid invoice, the unmown lawn, the lack of a mango.

People are parasites on the planet, they say, pointing out the reduced pollution in the big cities. The clear view of the Himalayan peaks is unprecedented in recent history.

Someone has to be really sick to resort to A&E. Everyone is staying away, they'd rather cope at home then come into that primordial stew of virus in the air.

Everyone has the right to be fearful, everyone has the right to complain.

You don't complain enough.

Are you enjoying this? The uncertainty, the gamble, the risk, all for the sake of helping others. You always wondered on what you based your claim to superiority, and now you have it.

You're selfish enough to put yourself last.

14

The Fridge

A couple of hours after writing the last entry, you wake up with an urgent pain in your gut. You feel hot and strange. You're still stubbornly camping downstairs in the living room, and find one of your ten-year-old twins is now beside you, snuffling comfortably. You slide out of bed, carefully, so as not to disturb her, and go to the toilet, in the dark.

Afterwards, you sit on the stairs and press your hands to your face. Your hands are always cold, it's a family joke that you could use them to chill wine. You suppose it's because your blood pressure is so low, what's normal for you would score two points in the early warning score for sepsis in the hospital. But now, your hands are worryingly warm. As warm as the little paws of the daughter taking over the double mattress with an imperial sprawl. Your nose is always cold, too. In those heat-sensitive imaging screens at the Science Museum, it always looks blue, a different climate to the rest of you. But it feels warm, too, even against your hot hands.

You've never, ever woken from sleep to go to the loo.

Diarrhoea is an early, lesser-known sign of Covid. Not many people know that. Most people know about fever and the rest of it.

You go back to bed. And when you wake, a few hours later, you feel fine. Your nose is as cold as your wine-cooler hands. You hug the children, do five hundred star jumps in front of the TV, while they lounge on the sofa and watch cartoons and mock you affectionately. You have to go to work half an hour earlier than your usual start time, for the ITU induction, and they protest that you haven't put their cereal on the table. You hug them again, and suggest, just once, they put it out for themselves. With some yoghurts and grapes from the fridge. It's cool outside, but you don't wear your cardigan. Instead you knot it around your neck as protection against the sun.

On the way to the ITU training, in the long corridor, you bump into the almost-consultant who is recruiting the new team into ITU. She asks if she should fight to have you on the definite-list, as you know the ITU so well. That means you're not on the definite-list, after all.

This is news to you. She explains that they've already picked ten doctors from the quietest non-medical wards, the Surgery and Obs and Gynae SHOs and juniors. The cancellation of clinics and elective surgeries means there are almost no patients for them. Whereas you have four bays and four side rooms needing your team's attention.

You don't know if you're disappointed or relieved. They don't need you now, but they're doubling the team, as they've doubled the beds from nine to eighteen.

It's predicted that at some point, they will need seventy ITU beds with ventilation support. She supposes that you'll be needed long before that happens.

You suppose you're relieved. Your colleague who'd messaged you isn't on the definite list either, and he is definitely relieved. His parents were terrified of him shifting onto ITU. And the ITU rota, as explained in the training, is punishing and democratic. Four and four and four for everyone. That means four days of twelve-hour shifts during the day. 8 a.m. to 8 p.m. Four days off. And then four sets of twelve-hour shifts through the night. 8 p.m. to 8 a.m.

Although you never get away at 8 a.m. after a night shift, and everyone knows that, as handover gets interrupted by emergency bleeps and slowed down by colleagues running late.

In the training you learn how to prone a patient, and you are taught the physiology of why it helps. No one calls it tummy time. It takes a lot of clinicians to do this safely, and ITU patients need to be turned regularly, this is one of the main reasons they need more doctors. You learn the physics behind the ventilated patient, and then they call out the names of the first ten to be transferred, who are starting the next day. The ten go to the ITU to be shown around. You go back to the ward and start preparing the notes to see your patients. No files or drug charts go in the bay anymore, no rolling computers, so everything must be looked up first, all the observations and blood results and imaging. And everything must be written up afterwards.

One of the team jobs is to write the death certificate of the patient who passed the morning before. The reg is the one who certified her death, and documented the cause of death, but he doesn't have the time to trek to the mortuary and sit in the bereavement office to fill out the small pile of paperwork. You agree to do it instead.

You go down to the hospital basement, to the mortuary offices, and they are more offhand with you than usual. They snap at you to sit down until they're ready. There is a Covid-positive patient they've had to get out of the fridge for the coroner, and they are a little stressed and fearful.

You've never really had to wait down there before. You sign the book confirming you're going to inspect the body of the patient, and look around, properly, for the first time. There is the large whiteboard with the names of the patients, and the number of the fridge space they've been allocated. There is another one of these, for the area around the corner. There is a smaller board you never noticed before. It says Perinatal Fridge.

Baby Jo. Baby Sam. Babies in the fridge.

You imagine what their mothers feel. If they knew that this cold, drab, officious place was where their babies were left. Bagged up like chicken.

Thank you, Doc, says the coroner to you, for no reason, as he leaves. You've done nothing helpful apart from keep out of the way. Perhaps our bar is now so low that keeping out of people's way is thoughtful and worthy of thanks. After all, getting close is now considered an act of aggression. Why did the chicken cross the road?

Because it was a considerate chicken.

You don't like it when people call you Doc. You think it's because they don't want to bother to look at your name badge. It's indifference hidden by a faux-respectful phrase. When you say Sister or Matron to a senior nurse, you say it with respect, with both syllables, and mean it.

And then you see the perinatal fridge. Tucked in the corner of the little anteroom that you normally sweep straight through to get into the office. About the size of those sofa-side beer fridges in American sitcoms. You're not sure if that's a lock on it. You have an urge to tug at it. You want to open it and check that Baby Jo and Baby Sam are OK.

You wonder what they dream in their frozen sleep. Their experiences of life must have been as bundled tight as they were in their respective wombs.

Shades of red and black.

Floating in warm fluid.

Tugging on a twisted umbilical cord like a plaything.

The voice they recognise, their mother's, talking in one tone to adults, and another tone to her bump. Her hand pressed protectively on her abdomen as they swim up to meet it, to press against it, or kick at it with their feet.

I'm here, they're saying. I'm still here.

You don't know if they ever took a breath before they went blue. You don't know if they ever saw light before they died, if they even blinked at the electric bulbs in the dun interiors of the labour suite. You don't know if they ever experienced the crushing violence of the contractions before they got wrapped up for the fridge.

There's a *Simpsons* joke, when Bart gets drunk and Marge wails that she's the worst mom in the world. And Homer says something like, No, she's not the worst, there's that freezer lady in Ohio.

We're ready, Doc, calls the mortuary assistant, giving you a strange look for hanging around at that bit of the office. He's probably wondering if you're going to steal from their stock of superior PPE in the unattended cupboards. They have those sturdier aprons.

Gown up, he says.

You pull on an apron, a mask and gloves, and go to see the patient.

You don't recognise this patient in death at all. Death doesn't become her. It doesn't complete her or perfect her. It's fed on her.

You don't know how death ever gets to be romanticised. She wasn't even sixty, but now she looks ancient, a carved statue lying on her own tomb in a church. You look at her tags and her bracelets, to confirm she is who she is. The protocol makes sense, as you don't really know her any more.

Then you gently press her chest for a pacemaker. They can explode in crematoriums. That's why you always check for one as part of the guidelines. It's what someone told you when you were a medical student, when you were first taught to examine bodies, and now that's what you tell other people whom you are instructing. One tiny detail in the sea of details you had to learn. You never asked how they explode or why they explode, and you never found out for yourself. You're not going to google it now.

When you complete the certification, back in the bereavement office, you notice the saddest thing. She was alone when she died. There was no family member, no friend there. You check again, hoping you're mistaken, leafing through the fat file of her medical notes, but you're not. You know that visitors have been banned from wards with Covid-positive patients. You know that even palliative patients' families are discouraged from coming.

Despite this, you know that her husband had been by her side since the end-of-life discussion was had. That was important to him and to her. But he wasn't there, that moment in the morning she passed away. He was probably brushing his teeth, getting shaved to look nice for her, packing some of her favourite treats into Tupperware. Anticipating a drowsy smile.

Ooh, my favourites, she might murmur, as she tries and fails to eats them.

He smiles, thinking about how surprised she'll be by the treats in the Tupperware, and he doesn't know that this moment of anticipation, of her slow grin spreading, of the wonder in her eyes, will be all he'll get. Just the anticipation. It won't happen. There will be no happy memory made. That's it.

She's lying cold in her fridge, in her whiteboard-allocated row and column of other bodies; and the lonely babies are in their own fridge at the exit or the entrance to this place, depending on your intentions.

You get another WhatsApp that all leave has been stopped, but you knew that. That the bank holidays will be cancelled. You knew that too. There had been the rumours from another site. You wait for an official email, a formal request, but it never comes. You get interrupted by another WhatsApp, asking if you'll be happy to do the 3/3/3 shift pattern, three days of 8 a.m. to 8 p.m., three days off, three nights of 8 p.m. to 8 a.m. You're not. There's another WhatsApp saying unfortunately the majority are happy so you'll need to do it too. It was never really a request. The third revised rota arrives and you don't bother to look at it, as it'll probably change tomorrow.

You will email the rota admin lead later, but there is a note that she is on holiday, and all emails sent while she is absent will be deleted on her return. It doesn't matter, anyway.

There are tears in your eyes, as you complete the cause of death paperwork. The window is open in the bereavement office, so maybe it is just your allergies, again. But the tears dripping freely make you feel sad, anyway, in the way that smiling makes you happier.

Progressive metastatic cancer. Breast, lung, bones, bowel, brain. The same cause of death someone would have written for your sister.

The days before she died, when she was no longer eating meals, and too drowsy on morphine to miss them, you brought her tidy brown-paper boxes of her favourite cake.

Pastel de nata. Custard in crispy pastry tarts, and she would lift them to her mouth in delight. Your anticipatory delight, that you had managed to do something right.

She could just press her lips to the pastry. Like an infant kiss. The sugared scent, the dry crisp of it. She couldn't take a bite. She couldn't swallow. And even if she could, her sluggish bowel could no longer digest. It would just sit there, like the guff and fluff at the bottom of a handbag.

This was never going to be a story with a happy ending.

Stories with happy endings are the ones that haven't finished yet.

15

Insider

It is day 18 of lockdown.

You're not working, the sunlight is streaming in through a gap in the curtains, the birds are chanting like schoolyard bullies, taunting all the people stuck inside while they swing freely in the sky, owning their space, like the straight couples who hog the pavement walking hand in hand. The seagulls huddle in menacing gangs like bikers, taking over garden walls. The sun is brutal. Everything has a brittle menace. The blue sky is like the cheap plastic bags in the pound shop. You've only had four hours' sleep because you were obsessively chronicling, scribing for your frontline tribe, sending aggrieved tweets and sad-scrolling through the Covid statistics.

There is so much to say, to process, to digest, that you can't take it all in at once. You can't understand the isolation memes and jokes, it's like everyone is talking a different language, with an If you don't laugh, you'll cry, Take *that*, Covid, captive jollity.

Have a cuppa, we're British.

Keep calm and carry on.

We'll meet again, said the Queen, on national TV.

And the language is back to the war.

He's a fighter.

You're a soldier.

They're heroes.

All the bombs are dropping.

Calm? War? It's all bollocks, isn't it?

And now you're not at work, with time to reflect, you're utterly humourless about it all.

Your life is on the line because of government incompetence.

Dozens of colleagues are dead because of government incompetence.

Thousands of people are dead because of government incompetence.

And they're not even giving the real figures, the uncounted ghosts missed out by the statistics.

You've written about the Eichmann trials. You've watched countless documentaries and read stories spun about genocide, euthanising whole societal demographics, decided upon by popular politicians flung into positions of power by public apathy and public relations spin.

You never thought it could happen to you, that it could happen here.

If a few pensioners die, so be it. Someone in the corridors of power said that, didn't they?

Did you really think that being British and middle class and educated would protect you? Did you really think you wouldn't get lined up against the wall with everyone else?

You didn't think that you would witness such loss, such horror, in your lifetime, in your country. And you never thought that were it to happen, no one would really care.

Almost a thousand people died yesterday, needlessly, on Good Friday, and the news outlets are mainly reporting that the prime minister gave a thankful wave as he left the hospital.

As though there were ever any possibility of him giving the finger and showing them his arse.

Yes, a clap and a wave might feel nice on Thursdays, but living another day, another week, making it to next Thursday, would be a bit nicer.

Didn't they vote against the nurses getting a pay rise, the cabinet, the whole stinking turd pile of them?

Didn't they just vote themselves an extra ten grand to sit at home on their tailored behinds?

The prime minister got it, and he beat it, they say.

The prime minister got it, it doesn't discriminate, they say.

Of course a virus doesn't discriminate.

People discriminate.

Who are the NHS workers, exposed and dying?

Who are the people living in cramped tower blocks?

Who are the vulnerable, living in care homes?

Who are the shopworkers, the delivery people, the key workers, the carers?

They quietly voted that these people, people who are keeping the country running, are the ones who will be scrutinised. Poorly paid and undervalued, and you don't get to stay in this country unless you're buried in it, six feet under, or until your dust is neatly funnelled into an urn.

The poor are the most exposed. The vulnerable are the most likely to die.

Thrown to the wolves. Cannon fodder.

There have been only four Covid deaths in New Zealand, a country with a population of five million, because they locked down early.

The two thousand people who died today and yesterday caught the virus before lockdown. When the government were putting their other concerns before human lives.

It's like they've put the population in a long conga line, and shot every hundredth person.

And they've always put someone old, someone weak, someone BAME or in healthcare in the hundredth spot.

You're angry. Not working gives you time to get angry. Your children think you are cranky because you're tired, and that's true too. You've still got the diarrhoea, and you are obsessively touching your hands, touching your cooler peripheries, trying to gauge if the temperature is coming, the spiking fever, the cough.

You checked the figures. You keep the screenshot of the stats on your phone like a talisman. Only half a per cent of people with the virus in your age bracket will die. Only.

That's at least five of your hospital colleagues.

Four of your graduating class.

Every single doctor who has died so far has been BAME.

There's a lot of stammering about how BAME people have diabetes anyway, or heart disease, how more of us are in the NHS. How the doctors who died were old, apart from the ones who weren't.

Do they use WAME in other countries, where the population is mainly not White? White and Minority Ethnic. You've never heard it if they do.

Every single dead doctor was brown or black.

Your family goes out and you stay in.

Your friends and relatives send you concerned and needy messages wanting you to tell them about what is going on.

Someone from the hospital is sending WhatsApp messages telling you that you will be working twelve-and-a-half-hour shifts every day, from 8.30 a.m. to

9 p.m., or 8.30 p.m. to 9 a.m. They don't say when but it is implied it will be immediate. They don't ask about childcare. Or well-being. Or whether you want to work those shifts. That's tomorrow's problem, when it'll be different.

No one has the right to demand this of you.

Your life for others.

Your time without consent.

Even that German cannibal asked consent before he ate his guest.

Your children come back from their allocated hour of outdoor exercise, wet, grumpy, sandy, flint in their feet. They feel uncomfortable outside now. Like they're off the map, and here there be dragons. They feel uncomfortable if they stop moving, when they're out, like they have become more of a target. The lockdown has made everyone a bit agoraphobic.

Your house is either a sanctuary or a prison, however you like to look at it.

Your house is not a lovely house.

But even heaven is a prison if you can't leave.

So, you're an insider now.

You're all insiders.

You all blow the whistle, again and again, and no one is listening. They know already, anyway. It's just that they don't care.

But there are chocolate eggs for the staff for Easter.

Keep calm and carry on.

You stop typing, as you can feel heat between the keys and your hands. Your hands feel warm. Too warm?

But it's a warm day.

Don't think about the dead, and those dying alone. Don't think about the masks being tugged and tied on and the files being handled with gloved hands. The death certification, again and again. The cool of the mortuary fridges. The babies waiting patiently, swaddled and gift-wrapped for God.

Isn't it a beautiful day? Aren't we so lucky to be alive? Today. Now. Air and water and sunshine and birdsong. An open window. Something is starting. With your warmed hands.

A sickness at your centre, spiralling out to your skin.

You're there, aren't you? Lining up like princesses at a party. Gowned. Crowned. Waiting for your big entrance.

You're all inside, looking out.

16
Nostradamus

It's day 20 of lockdown, and you can't understand the lack of anger in the newspapers, in the news outlets, on the television.

You don't understand how 10,000 dead isn't written in big, blood-red letters everywhere.

You don't understand how 10,000 preventable deaths hasn't toppled the government, caused a revolution, caused CHANGE.

Facts are unimportant, it seems. The fact of 10,000 lives lost. Their names should be printed in waves down every front page, on every splash page of the internet, but instead they are dismissed as a statistic before the bodies are even buried. Her gran, his nan, her dad, his son. Our loved one. Unacknowledged.

And the sinking, creeping fear that these 10,000 are just the start. That it may be 100,000 before this is over.

The virus isn't the villain of the piece. It's the politicians.

You used to say, cynically, that brown and black lives lost weren't important to the West. You were talking about famine and natural disasters in distant parts of

Africa and Asia. The floods in Bangladesh, where your mother grew up.

But now, you realise, it's not ethnicity or distance that causes indifference. It's the lives themselves. Other people's lives aren't important to people of power and privilege in the West.

Not the old, not the vulnerable.

The people of power and privilege only care about their own lives. Their lives, their rules.

This is a crime. This is criminal negligence. And however many times you all say it, and it echoes around the internet, no one appears to be listening.

The internet is more interested in joking about Priti Patel's eyebrows than her errors. They ask, How did she get them done so neatly in lockdown? You want to ask, How come she can't count?

The newspapers and news channels are more interested in making tributes to dead celebrities. A comedian. A racing driver. And reporting some heart-warming stories about key workers dancing with their colleagues, without acknowledging their fear and forced sacrifice of personal safety.

Instead of being accused, the government become accusers of those they are meant to be protecting. They say, Don't waste the PPE, it's a valuable resource.

More valuable than the lives of those caring for the Covid patients, and by extension, the lives of their own isolated families.

They say, I'm sorry if you feel that way.

There is no if. We do feel that way. That's why they need to apologise in the first place.

And what of the dead doctors and nurses?

They say, We don't know they caught Covid looking after patients. They could have caught it on the bus.

So it seems that we, the doctors, are accused of wastefulness, of complaining, of resentment, and of carelessness.

And those are just the bits you remember before you switch off the screen in frustration.

10,000 names on a list. 10,000 people calling out to be remembered, for their deaths not to have been useless.

You're falling asleep as you write into the night. You're writing on the floor, as your desk is now taken over by Lego projects and home-schooling exercise books and scattered homework printouts and coloured pens.

Someone said that Nostradamus had predicted a lung disease that would be transmittable in 2020. People like you are bleating like Cassandra about the dire consequences, and they are ignored.

Young doctors are already so normalised to this new version of reality that they unfriend and bitch about any medic who takes time off due to fearfulness or anxiety. Medical Twitter laughs at the attention-seeking colleagues who take selfies gowned up in full PPE like Darth Vader, who solicit new likes and a Hero nickname with exaggeration of their roles, with bragging posts of their selfless redeployment to A&E. Like it is some sort of reality show that they are watching and playing and winning.

They are without fear, and this makes sense to you.

You can't live with fear.

But you can try to live without it.

Everyone else's concerns, in the family and friends circle and the wider world, seem increasingly irrelevant and indulgent to you.

Running out of gift wrap, and being forced to substitute Christmas wrap instead.

Coffee beans being delivered instead of ground coffee.

Ranting about purchase orders. Bad reviews on social media. Home haircuts. Roots showing on their dye jobs.

You've woken up on your laptop again. A line of characters like cartoon-swearing streaming out under your chin and on to your screen.

The morning is wiser than the evening. It will make more sense in the morning.

17

Resurrection

Day 21 of lockdown, and reading the papers, watching the news, you'd think only one person had been seriously ill, and that he, thanks to the well-staffed and well-supplied NHS, had got better. The newsreader has obviously done her own hair and make-up, which is a nice touch.

There are only feel-good stories, which is disconcerting. The postie doing his rounds in fancy dress. The trucker determinedly delivering potatoes. The school open over the Easter bank holiday.

You flick to another news programme, as you feel certain you must have blinked and missed it. The 10,000 dead, fire and fury and… no, you didn't miss it. It wasn't there.

The PM is thanking the ITU nurses who looked after him. They're both from abroad.

You wonder what conversations they had, as they remained by his bedside, day and night, not leaving him unattended for even a minute to get a fresh syringe, without getting someone else to take their watchful place. They would have probably talked about hospital breakfast, the weather. Maybe they talked about their long shifts in Intensive Care, their specialised training, their fears. You wonder if he told them why he voted against a pay rise for nurses, along with most of the current cabinet. You wonder if he told how he voted at all.

His partner is tearfully saying she can't possibly thank the NHS enough, that no one can.

You and everyone else is thinking, well, *he* can. He can freaking start with the figure of millions he painted down the side of a bus. He's probably already planning his Survival Memoir, and talking to his publishing cronics about the advance.

Cynically, being ill has done him no harm. Like the Queen Mother getting bombed in Buckingham Palace during the war. She said she could finally look the East End in the face.

It's made him one of the many.

The duty of the free press is to the governed, not the governors.

You realise that perhaps you're not free. It's just been an illusion. Perhaps you really are all cast in some endless Truman show. The death toll isn't real, it is just a number ticking and increasing, the views swelling on Twitter.

Your child asks you if Jesus was meant to have risen on Easter Sunday or Monday. You can't remember.

The PM has risen over Easter, and you think that he has managed to get away with it, after all.

Get away with an illness that has killed many younger and fitter than him.

Get away with this loss and horror on his watch.

He doesn't seem particularly bright, so it must just be luck. Some people are luckier than others. You're a gambler's daughter, you know something about the power of outrageous fortune.

You finally look at your phone, and see several messages from work. They think you're on the A&E team. You tell them you're not. You resend the email to work, explaining why you couldn't work today, on the bank holiday. You see that every other doctor has been called into the hospital, but many have no role at all, and are not scheduled on any particular ward, so are sitting listlessly in the mess, or asking the wards to message if they are needed. You say you'll be in tomorrow. But you have that diarrhoea again and now you have a rash. Viral exanthem? Another little-known sign of Covid infection. It's been over a week since you were most clearly exposed. That countdown.

You're feeling guilty for not calling your mother. But nothing you say to her will reassure her. And she always tells you that you're looking sick.

When your sister died, with all the planning and preparation, the counselling and the memory boxes, the hospice vigil, you never thought that you would be the next one in line.

No preparation. No counselling. No memory boxes for the kids. When you mention a funeral, casually, the children ask you which cakes you'd like served. They say that they know cake is important to you, and they don't want to mess that up.

Heartless, pragmatic little munchkins. Fearless.

Your sister would be pretty fucked off to see you there so soon, as an NHS martyr. Showing her up, and stealing her thunder.

Go away, she hisses at you, you're here forty years too early!

What about him, you say, nodding at your dad, manspreading in the armchair in the corner. Reading the *Racing Post* or something equally unlikely in the Muslim heavenly garden.

Him? He was here forty years too late, she scoffs.

I shouldn't be here at all, you point out. Everyone knows you're not much of a believer. She was a believer for ages, it turns out, but kept it on the down-low.

Oh that, she shrugs. It's not like you've got a choice. You gotta be good if you're dead.

You wrote that line, when she was dying. It was in her poem. You're touched she remembers.

You go back. The 10,000 stream over you, unfurling like ribbons, wisps of satin shadow, flowing past your fingers like cool water.

You're not one of them.

You're no martyr.

You're not good or dead.

Fewer deaths today. It might be weekend under-reporting. It might be that those who caught it before lockdown are either better or have already passed. People coming into hospital now must be post-lockdown, as three weeks is the longest it might take to present.

More messages. The rota will change. Not the 3/3/3 they threatened. Three twelve-hour day shifts, three twelve-hour night shifts, three days off, repeat. Something else. They'll know tomorrow. Maybe the next day.

You pick at the rash on your arm.

Your daughter picks up the hat you used to wear to work, realises what it is, and drops it like it's diseased. She assiduously washes her hands.

You should have called your mother.

You can't tell her about the deaths, the new diagnoses, about the vomiting patient and the consultants you work with who are now Covid positive. You can't tell her about the rota changing. The messages screeching from your phone. The uncertainty.

You do some admin emails. Write the mandatory reflective piece for your medical training portfolio. Invoice the University of Oxford for your masters workshops.

You make apple crumble. You make dinner. You watch the children playing and give them a thumbs-up whenever they look at you for approval.

You play them at chess, and try hard to win, and when it's within your grasp, you make an imperfect but plausible move, so they win instead, and are convinced it's deserved. That you didn't just let them.

Your children's father is howling with laughter and clapping his hands at something streaming on his tablet from the top room.

You fiddle with your sister's faded flowers at the corner of the kitchen table, where her condolence cards are still concertinaed together. Easter Monday.

You tell your sister about the prime minister's miraculous turn in ITU, already home and heading for the country, shedding his viral load from the speeding car like confetti blown on the wind.

A resurrection, you tell her. When you heard he was heading to ITU, you supposed he'd be ventilated, and then he'd be dead. And you supposed his prognosis would be that poor as he looks like a vasculopath with metabolic syndrome, stacked up with stiff arteries, fatty liver and pre-diabetes. There are already rumours that he wasn't as sick as he implied, that he might not have had Covid at all.

If you're feeling dramatic, you joke to your sister, it would be a great day for another resurrection. If you fancied upstaging someone. Everyone's doing it today. A blond fraud out of ITU. The OP coming out of a cave. She doesn't dignify that one with a response. You think she's there, but giving you the silent treatment. You just about catch an offended huff, over the B-flat background hum. You forgot she'd caught religion.

You should call your mum. She's lost one daughter and now she's worried for another. I'm fine, you should say, just fine. It's going to be all right.

But you don't want to reassure her falsely. You can't.

18

Rage

Day 22 of lockdown, and at 6 a.m. your children are catastrophising disaster scenarios where there's no water, no food, no electricity, no Wi-Fi.

You're lucky that you live in England, you say, you can always collect rainwater. It's probably cleaner now than it's been in years.

You're lucky we live by the sea. We can fish.

You can build a wind turbine, you say. Like the kid in that movie who saved his village and irrigated the fields, with a textbook and a bike wheel.

You draw a blank at cup-half-full suggestions about the Wi-Fi. You tell them when the online games are over, they can read all the books littering the house, and when those are finished, they can all write some more, and if the children don't want that, they can paint and play music and embroider cushion covers like nineteenth-century ladies of accomplishment. They are unimpressed and tell you that you're being sexist.

The teenagers are watching a movie about a pandemic that is mildly worse than this one. The photogenic scientists seem to kill a lot of monkeys, but they get to a cure by day 30. People seem to care in the movies about a fictional killer virus a lot more than they do in real life. There's rioting and tears and government inquiries and pharmacies are trashed and for some inexplicable reason there appears to be a shortage of blankets for shivering patients, who are forced to borrow coats instead. They run out of body bags, they rob houses for food and guns.

At least they all have PPE, you think humourlessly, watching the gangs stalking the streets in masks, with hoods and full suits.

No one behaves like that, now we're in the fiction, staring from the other side of the mirror, on the inside of the screen. The 1 per cent shrugs and dies obligingly, like it's impolite to do otherwise, because they don't want to be a strain on the health services. Everyone else says stiff-upper-lip stuff, like they're trying their best. Like they don't believe they'd let us die. Except they have and they will. They've let healthy thirteen-year-old children and thirty-something mothers die, they've let dedicated doctors die, doctors who put themselves out to help.

They don't say what they see, maybe it's just too horrible. Easier to say what they want to see.

In the movie, no one is working apart from the government researchers in their sealed monkey-murdering facility. The police and the doctors aren't turning up to their jobs. They're too scared of the infection.

In the real world, you turn up to work, along with everyone else. A registrar is there, who doesn't want to be at the hospital, and is honest and vocal about it. The consultants complain about this colleague, saying things like, You can see someone's true character in a crisis.

That's not true, it's not their true character. No one is themselves in a crisis.

You feel sweaty and chilly all the long walk to work. The viral exanthem, that persistent rash, bubbling along your arms. At the hospital you ask one of the linen suppliers for scrubs, as you know your ward doesn't carry any your size. They say no. You go to the ward and see everyone is in mismatched and ill-fitting scrubs, even the ward manager. You ask them to take your temperature, as it is exactly a week since you were in a car with your Covid-positive consultant. You're 36 degrees, on the cold side of normal.

You're reassured, at least. You find scrubs the size of a sail. You start to prepare the ward round.

The patients who are extubated from ITU, recovering from Covid.

A patient having a heart attack.

A dying patient crying about her DNACPR form which was completed on her admission in the Emergency Department. Insisting she won't sign. Shocked that it doesn't need her signature, it's the lead doctor's decision, not the patient's. American TV has misled her about that.

A patient who is deaf, dumb and blind.

A patient who spits at you not to touch her, when you examine the healthy arm she insists is broken.

A patient who is starting biologic treatment at £10,000 a year, which won't cost her family a penny, but who might die, anyway.

A patient who has not been given anticoagulant medication for three days because of fear about her anaemic haemoglobin level, who is now having a pulmonary embolism, a clot in her lungs.

A patient who is deceptively healthy, annoyed to be admitted, whose care has been mismanaged for a year in another Trust.

It's a good day, because no one dies. There are no new Covid cases on your ward.

A partial rota is issued for two of the Covid bays, and everyone else in medicine wonders whether they should even go in tomorrow, as they don't have a rota at all.

A patient is concerned about a failed procedure, and you go and speak to her about it. You are already thirty minutes late.

You're leaving the ward when you hear the sister complaining about how someone wrote IV medication for a new patient without putting in a cannula.

You walk back and admit it was you, and apologise, and go to do that.

She stops you, as you've already changed into day clothes, and shouldn't be on the ward.

You leave late, but still feel guilty.

When you get home, you just want to eat and sleep. The children fall asleep around you. Purring like kittens.

You're not watching the news, but the normality of the day impresses itself.

The extubated patients are getting better.

No new Covid diagnoses or deaths on the ward.

You don't know what happened at the end of that virus film. Maybe someone went to jail for profiteering. Maybe someone won the Nobel for the cure.

Maybe a lot more people died. But quietly.

You should say nothing. You should talk to no one.

You should say everything. Shout it out into the crowded night. Rage.

Thousands of dead and dying. Dying quietly, counted daily. Dylan Thomas wrote about his dying father, an echoing villanelle titled, Do not go gentle into that good night. He was right.

They should not go so gently.

19
Mothers

Your ward is suddenly overstaffed for the day. You're not sure why, perhaps the surgical teams and community teams have been added to the medical rota. It's not much more helpful than being understaffed. The extra doctors loll about on their phones, as they don't know the patients, only one or two of you can enter the bays for the ward round and there is limited work that can be done without a computer, and there are still only three of those on the long desk.

Without a computer, you can't check the blood results. You can't order them, either.

You can't look at imaging, like X-rays and CT scans and MRIs and ultrasounds, and you can't read the reports.

You can't check the patient observations, to see who spiked a temperature, whose ulcerative colitis is producing explosive bowel movements, whose blood pressure is dangerously low.

You can't go into the patient records, to see their baseline function, their old appointments and letters, their medical history.

You can't see their usual prescription medication to complete their drug chart.

You can't refer to colleagues, or see how the specialities have responded.

You can't discharge patients, or book their ongoing outpatient investigations.

All you can do without the computer is examine the patients. Or do procedures.

The spare doctors aren't doing this, either. You just carry on and do your job, and you don't delegate.

The trouble with having too many people about is that no one is taking responsibility for that bay, that side room, that patient. It's the same problem across the hospital, when all the junior doctors on the other wards seem to finish at 5 p.m. on the dot and dozens of reallocated doctors crowd out the medical wards, asking if there's anything they can do. They end up in the mess by midday, eating the free sandwiches. Disconsolately. It's better to be busy, to be useful, than to be bored.

The national news is about a nurse who had died in her third trimester. Her baby was saved by C-section. You wonder if her little girl will ever forgive the architects of this tragedy. You wonder if she'll be the one to grow up and make something right.

On the ward, there's a mother who has exhausted all the curative options for her disease. None of them have helped. She is now for palliative care only. She knows this. She has suspected it for some time. You ask if she wants you there when she talks to her family. She is more worried for her two grown-up daughters than she is for herself.

I have two daughters, too, you say. She smiles at you, for sharing this.

They're everything, aren't they, she says.

20

Sad Face

You're utterly humourless about this situation, and it shows.

You're living with low-level fear every day, and it causes your skin to break out, your allergies to stream out of your eyes and nose, and your mood to pool around your boots.

You're constantly on edge. You can't physically sit down, unless you collapse to sleep. It weirds out your colleagues.

You dress at your front door, so your work clothes and shoes and jacket aren't contaminating the house.

You walk to work every day, aware of every sniffle and cough.

You make up stories on your way, of why you haven't made it in, why you've had to call it a day. Why you can't go on. You go on, anyway.

No one thought of anything as horrible as this when they decided to train to be a doctor. You've got kids. Why are you punishing yourself?

They need you. You need you.

You haven't planned a funeral. You haven't made a will. You're glad your children are unsentimental, that they have so much backup, with each other, that they are used to your absence at work every day. At least they've got your books to read, although they've never shown much interest in them, not even to be polite. They're refreshingly free from diplomacy, and you envy them that freedom. They can turn down any invitation with a casual, No thanks, I don't really want to, it sounds kind of noobish, and suffer no agonies of guilt. When you point out that they really should – It's her birthday! It's a funeral! It's Eid! It's my book and it's dedicated to you! It's your friend and you promised! – it does nothing.

They just roll their eyes like some collective organism, a social swarming being of buzzing bees, and say, Guilt-tripping? Really? So uncool. They say it ironically, like it's a joke you're sharing. And you admire both the timing and the ability to deliver a line with just the right pitch of low-level disappointment and outrage.

You haven't told them where you buried the cursed pirate treasure. The codes to activate the robot army. You haven't given them the map with an X to mark the spot. Now *that* they'd be interested in.

You're making up symptoms, on your long walk lined with bushes and brambles and fields, you're dissembling so well you fool yourself. You're hot, you're practically sweating. Your hands are so cold, you must be shutting down peripherally. Is that a cough? Is that a dry cough? Can you smell the flowers? You're not sure you can smell them. You'll need to mask up and leave the moment you get to the ward. You'll need to tell them.

You get into the ward, and stop at the nurse's station, and ask them to take your temperature, again. You feel sweaty and shaking, and you'd been coughing all the way there. Everyone's allergies are horrible this year, and yours are playing up. Your temperature is only 36.7 degrees. You're afebrile. Once you know you're OK, you don't cough again. Maybe you really were making it up. You change into scrubs and start the day.

All day at work, people say things like, Why so sad? Why so serious, Doctor? Why the long face?, like you're a horse who's walked into a bar. It feels like every workman on every building site you've ever walked past as a teenager is talking to you.

You don't take exception. It is working women who are asking. Nursing staff and colleagues. Maybe you smile too much on ordinary days, you had smile lines by the time you were eighteen. You've always known you have the sort of face that looks miserable in repose.

When other people make jokes about getting the last ventilator, drafting their own will, gifting their belongings, you're not laughing.

The PPE has been downgraded, due to availability, and a colleague on the Covid ward, who should have been in a proper gown, had blood spray across her skin during a procedure.

She carries on and completes it.

You all keep calm and carry on.

21

Sputter and Gag

It's the twenty-fifth day of lockdown.

The nursing colleague who said, Why the long face, is now feeling poorly. They ask you to swab her nose and throat. She is the one who is trained to do it, she is the one who has swabbed the most difficult patients for the virus, and has done it pragmatically, without complaint or excuse. The deaf and blind patient, nearing end of life due to a rare disease, and you can't even explain what has happened to her. The schizophrenic patient who is now ten days behind on her depot psych medication, something you unearthed when you dug deeper, just because you took it personally when she snapped, Don't touch me! as she turned her face to the wall like a sixty-year-old teenager. The patient with cancer. The patient who is immunosuppressed, with bowel disease that will kill her before the virus.

This nurse is the one who puts on a surgical mask, an apron and gloves, which is all you are issued as full PPE for these patients who might be positive, and puts the swab deep in their nose, until their eyes water, and they sneeze; and then she puts another swab deep in their throat, until they cough and gag at you. She does it properly. She takes that risk.

And now she has a temperature. She has a cough. And they ask you to swab her nose and her throat.

You realise that when she said, Why the long face? that she meant it. It wasn't an insult. It was concern. When you feel sad, and serious and sick in yourself, you recognise it in others.

You used to pride yourself on being the helpful doctor in the office, the one who takes the time to bleed the patient for that test, when the others are having tea or checking their phones or updating their portfolios or bonding with the boss, the one who drags out the ultrasound machine to cannulate a difficult patient when the nurses are struggling, the one who comes straight out to review the patient the nurses are worried about. The one who avoids someone having to say, Well don't all jump at once, when something routine has been requested, and the others are staring at screens and avoiding eye contact.

That's why they asked you, the most junior doctor, first. The other doctors in the room don't think you're helpful, they just think you're a bit of a sucker. You're the oddity. The non-career doctor. The one who doesn't really need the job. That's usually forgotten when you're all getting on with your tasks, but sometimes they're reminded of it.

You don't help this time. Instead, you look helplessly around at the three other doctors in the office, who are all senior to you by several years. A senior house officer, a core trainee, a senior registrar. The SHO is actually a senior SHO, which seems to be making too much of a point of the seniority.

Do you know how to do a Covid swab? you ask them. I've never done one.

This is true. You've not even seen one done. Previously, they've been done in closed rooms by someone with full PPE, and you are told not to waste it. So unless you are in the room, too, you don't wear it. You certainly don't waste a set just to watch someone swab.

No, says the core trainee. No, says the senior SHO. No, says the reg.

Have you at least seen it done? you ask.

No, No, No. You suppose that at least one of them is lying. You're four weeks into the pandemic.

There are two senior nurses in the room, who have been specialists in Intensive Care and mental health, but are now helping out on the wards.

I know the theory, they say. One of them explains it, and she has seen it done. She describes poking it painfully deep until you get the sputtering cough and gagging.

You all know the theory. You have all taken swabs many times before. But just not for this. Another experienced nurse turns up and goes to do it herself, and the doctors sigh collectively with relief.

You feel dirty and dishonest, even though you didn't lie.

The reason you didn't want to do it wasn't because you'd never seen one done before. That wouldn't have stopped you, rightly or wrongly, as a lot of the job is learned by doing. The reason you didn't want to do it wasn't because of the infection risk, although you are guessing that is what stopped your colleagues.

It was because you didn't want to be responsible for doing it wrong. For not going deep enough in the nose, in the throat. For not making the eyes water and the nurse gag. Because if you do it wrong, and you don't cause the pain, cause the hurt, it will come back falsely negative.

And she'll be back at work in two days, falsely reassured, spreading the virus around like canapés at a party.

You're paralysed. You can't do the most straightforward and necessary job at this strange time. One that patients could do themselves if they were keen. You can't do the test to diagnose the virus.

What use are you, really? What use are any of you?

Avoiding the trivial jobs of great importance suddenly seems to be another disease you can catch, as you feel uncertain you have any skills at all.

You avoid clerking a patient.

You avoid placing a cannula.

When a patient desaturates, you avoid taking a further blood gas, and chase up the respiratory team instead.

It's not just you. All the doctors feel that way. There are too many of you about now, to feel the usual accountability. Doctors and nurses, who are meant to be on annual leave, are on the wards. All the speciality doctors and nurses have been redeployed. You've divided up the ward, taking care of your patients, avoiding questions about the others, because you know nothing about them. You go to the mess to toast your sandwich, and find it full of doctors lolling on the wipe-clean plastic sofas. You don't recognise most of them.

You should ask for help, when you're busy, says one you do know. Some of these guys have been here since 11 a.m. with nothing to do.

We're doing our own rota, says another, We're just leaving the wards with too many doctors, and going to the other ones.

It's stupid, says another, No one would know if I was here or not. I've been called over from the other hospital, and nobody knows who I am or what I'm meant to be doing, or where.

At least you've got a base ward, says someone else to you. You know where to go in the morning.

I was driving in, and got told at 8.30 a.m. to take a zero day, to head back home, as they're gonna put me on call tomorrow.

The seniors on surgery and specialities have no juniors, and fed up with taking their own bloods and doing their own clerking, try to pass over their patients to the medical wards. It's like if they're not cutting into someone, they don't know what to do, says a medical consultant, not even joking.

The juniors who have been shifted onto medicine have no rota. No base ward to go to in the morning. No continuity of patient care or supervision. It's unsafe for everybody. They talk about a rota, but nothing comes. One ward, the ward dealing exclusively with Covid-positive patients, has a rota, to rotate those wearing full PPE for long shifts, and that is it.

And then the question about full PPE. The guidelines change based on availability, and Covid-19 has quietly been downgraded to a less serious pandemic than SARS, despite the 1,000 dying every day. The entire SARS outbreak took 780 lives. And the full PPE has been downgraded to the plastic pinny, a surgical mask and regular examination gloves. No sleeves. A doctor talks about taking bloods from a Covid-positive patient, how she grabbed his bare arm instinctively. He couldn't wash it while in the bay; everything else is potentially loaded with virus.

Another doctor says that the masks don't stop anything reaching the back of your throat. Rather, they stop you coughing on people. It's the patients who should wear them, not the doctors.

The FFP masks, which offer better protection, have been taken off every ward without patients who are confirmed Covid-positive by lab test. Which means that every time you swab someone, they are shifted to a different bay, a Covid-positive one, as that is the only place with the masks.

A matron from the Covid-positive ward turns up and accuses your consultant of swabbing people just to lighten his own workload. It's the end of the day, and everyone is on edge.

You see that after all your bitching about the PPE decision from managers, NHS communications have asked to use a smiling photo of you in scrubs tweeted by your publisher. Of course, you reply, quietly. Embarrassed by the attention. Thank you for asking.

It doesn't feel like you're all in this together. It feels more like you're puppies being shepherded uselessly about, bouncing around a closed space.

You don't think you did any harm.

But you don't think you saved anyone. Apart from the healthy ones who you are safely discharging as quickly as you can, before they get sick in hospital, too.

The death toll of the BAME doctors is rising. It's still every dead doctor. All aged forty plus. But you know you'll survive it, when you get it.

At least you know that much. You are less useful dead than alive.

How many others are being given that reassurance?

22

Sick

It's almost the fourth week of lockdown. Day 26.

A few days ago you were asked for access to your sick records. Not an official request, but one made by WhatsApp. You replied that they had your permission, but added, with a slightly aggrieved tone, that you didn't think you'd had any sick days. That's something you pride yourself on. Your stubborn constitution. You're never ill, and you have always had a sneaking old-school suspicion that people who take sick days are frauds. And your body can put up with pain.

When you were a child, seven years old, you'd had appendicitis for a week before you admitted you had a stomach ache to your mother. And only then because she'd challenged you, seeing you crouching about your room, bent over. When they cut into you, your appendix was so swollen it was fit to burst. They told your mother that you'd escaped peritonitis by a few hours.

When you were expecting your second baby, you mistook labour pains for hunger, and read magazines in the bath, eating a box of chocolates, before you realised what they were. You were far too late to the hospital to have the epidural that had been planned. They said you were lucky not to have popped the baby out in the car.

There was a WhatsApp reply. It's not for sick days you've taken, they said, it's for the sick days you're going to take. As though it were inevitable.

You're a bit offended. You're not one of those, constantly whining about bad backs and coughs and colds.

You complain about the assumption in the mess, to someone who had been off sick, but had been called back in, as her test was Covid negative. She said she still felt poorly, but had been forced to return. Against the guidelines of the full seven days off, as she'd been forty-eight hours without a fever.

One of those. You don't think she's that sick. You don't move away from her.

On the Sunday morning, you wake feeling hot and cold. One of your children is hugging you, and they notice that your hands are warm instead of cool. You've already said how that's unusual for you. Feverish patients usually sigh with relief when you examine them. Others jump at your touch, with a Christ-that's-cold! Cold hands warm heart, they add, as though concerned that they might have offended you.

Your resting blood pressure is ninety over sixty, which would grade you for a sepsis early warning score. Your usual temperature is 36 degrees, which would give you another point. Warm hands are not a sign of comfort for you, and in your instance are not reassuring. They are a sign of fever.

During the day, a non-strenuous Sunday, watching TV, in the bath with the kids, sitting in the garden, putting out oven-baked food, making cupcakes, you feel stretched, and your nerves feel jangled. You feel sore and tired and floppy and irritable. Everything is conspiring to irritate you. The beauty of the day. The plastic blue sky. The swept garden. The children's fierce laughter. The screeching of the fearless birds. The children are doing something complicated on an online game that involves them checking in every few minutes, when they are meant to be outside and screen-free, just for the hour after lunch. They ignore you, scenting your weakness, like sharks. You yell at them, and then tell them to do whatever they want. Your grumpiness and their guilt. So it feels that no one has won, and you have all lost. You abandon the cupcakes in the oven and stomp off.

You relent only when you smell the cakes, warm vanilla fog filling the rooms, and return to yank the tray out and dump it on the side, so they won't burn. You're cross but you won't waste food. Not just for a gesture.

You go upstairs, and collapse on the floor beside the bed. Your bones tugged down by gravity. You're just a bag of organs pooling to the ground. You hear the children coming up the stairs, apologising, talking to you, and you don't really register. You think they're asking for permission to do something. To carry on with their complicated game? Just answering a question feels complicated to you right now.

Just do what you want, you say.

This is their moment to profit from their misbehaviour. They could ask you for anything, and you'd say yes. They wouldn't even have to explain to their father, because Mum-said-we-could is the get-out-free card at the weekend. Ask anything.

Screens all night.

The chocolate egg stash.

The new game update.

The 15-rated programme.

The slide down the stairs in a box competition.

What they are actually asking you is this: Can we ice the cupcakes?

They repeat it a few times before you get it.

You're surprised they know how to ice cupcakes. They always let you do it, and then they just add a few flourishes after you're done, another squirt of colour, another dash of sprinkles.

An hour later, you're still dozing, and a cupcake is brought up to you. Two cupcakes, in fact. You're unbearably touched by how pretty they are. The generosity of the icing, the sprinkles more heavy-handed and varied than you would do yourself. Every jar of sprinkles you have has been put to use – the multi-coloured strands, the hundreds and thousands, the pearl-pastel balls, holly berries and holly leaves from Christmas.

You're still on the floor. You haven't even made it up to the bed. Your proximal muscles ache from the inside out. Your thighs, your upper arms. Your head swims when you lift it, and droops like it is weighed down. Snowdrops and narcissi, staring at the earth or their own reflection. Your eyes are hot in your head.

Daddy says you're tired and grumpy because you've been working through an unprecedented global pandemic, says one.

We thought you were just being mean, says another, cheerfully.

I am mean, you agree, making a fuss about the cupcake, without the appetite to eat more than a bite. You don't like excuses being made for you.

You've slept through the family Zoom call, but no one asks you why.

You're relieved not to be pestered. You're annoyed that no one asks where you were.

It's your turn to make dinner and you phone it in. You put frozen fish fingers and garlic bread on a tray, put it in the oven, and serve it with sliced fruit and raw vegetable sticks and ketchup. You put dinner on the picnic bench in the garden so you don't have to clean up crumbs.

You finally take your temperature again, and it is 38 degrees. For you, that's shockingly high. 2 degrees above your baseline. It's like 39 degrees for other people. You could wash clothes at that temperature. Hand-hot, is what they used to call it. That makes sense. Your hands are hot.

Your head is swimming, and you crawl into bed in your clothes. Not into bed. Onto the mattress where you were playing camp-out, in the living room. You tell your children not to hug you goodnight, not to get in the covers with you in the morning. You wake in the early evening with your clothes drenched in sweat, so you take them off. You wake again with your second T-shirt soaking, so you change it. It happens again. And again.

You finally admit it. You message your ward colleagues. I don't think I can come in tomorrow.

I think I'm sick.

You're one of those. You're just a number after all.

23

The Good Death

It's day 27 of lockdown.

You tell work what happened to you the day before, you apologise to your family and your friends whom you virtually stood up. Had a raging fever, you say, muscle-achey, floppy, head-achey.

But this morning, you feel like a fraud. Now you can get up and make tea, and watch TV. You could work. But it's too late to deny that you were sick, and it would be too irresponsible to ignore how you felt on that sunny Sunday. Your rota coordinator has already told you to isolate for seven days and to get tested. You book it for the next day, and are surprised how easy it is to do.

You have no chest symptoms. No cough. No shortness of breath. No sore throat. No anosmia. You're sure it's not Covid. You're sure.

You've got something, though. Viral, definitely. Your lymph nodes are raised.

Your whole family can't go out until you get a negative test. If you're positive, they're stuck indoors for fourteen days. They couldn't care less. They have biscuits and ice cream and crisps and chocolate and Wi-Fi. They have yesterday's extravagantly iced cupcakes.

When you went hiking for Duke of Edinburgh, as a teenager, all you brought with you were two maxi packets of mini Mars bars. Your teammates thought you were a hero. That's all you ate, apart from milk scavenged from a farm.

You tell the children to keep away from you, and they try. You stay buried under your duvet, in your living room, like a troll under a bridge. You thought they'd be terrified of you, if you were ill. You'd feel a bit more reassured if they were. Instead, they make jokes about social distance and about your lurgies.

Messages start coming through. How someone else who was positive had no chest symptoms. How that only happened one week after onset.

You still don't think you have it, and you doubt it would be picked up if you do. And you know how unreliable the test is. It was why you were so fearful of doing it. If you just do a painless tickle around the nostrils and the tonsils, there's no chance of any detectable virus, you have to go high, you have to go deep.

And the test is drive-through, through a window, they're not going to go deep, they don't want you sneezing and coughing on them. You'll be clear in two days, and back at work. Passing around your infection.

But that fever keeps spiking. You keep getting shakes and sweats. You wonder if you have endocarditis or influenza A, before you reflect that those really are not better options.

What if it's not viral? Some days ago, you took blood from a patient's PICC line, pulled the dark venous blood out with a long syringe with sterile gloves. And when you were filling the various bottles in the clinical room, the yellow bottle for electrolytes, the blue for clotting, the purple for the full blood count, the blood suddenly sprayed across the open wounds on your arm. From that unresolved rash of unknown origin.

You check the patient's results, and confirm that the patient didn't have a bacteraemia. You know some viruses can sit in blood. Even Covid can. You remember that the wounds were inflamed two days after. They're scabbing over nicely, now.

You sit at home feeling useless. You find out that lots of other doctors your grade have been off work, too. Because someone in their flat had a temperature, so they all have to stay at home. The hospital probably thinks you're all malingering.

The on-call team is pleading for junior doctors on the group WhatsApp. Too many have become too few again.

The management responds. They insist that those doctors in affected households should come in if they're asymptomatic, saying it was confirmed as acceptable by the virologist. After all, the doctors' communal housing has separate bedrooms and bathrooms. Shared space notwithstanding.

This new directive is against national guidelines. No doctor from an affected flat, with an affected housemate, wants to go in the hospital and risk killing patients as an asymptomatic carrier. The decision by management is challenged, and reversed a few hours later, probably when the virologists realised what they had signed their name to, being the named clinicians responsible for sending young doctors from Covid-query households back to vulnerable patients on the wards and A&E. To be fair, the virologists were from a different part of the Trust, where the doctors' accommodation is a single-cell room, with no communal areas. They didn't realise the doctors in your hospital share a kitchen and living room.

The only two doctors who had been successfully hounded into going into the hospital are sent back home. It turns out that there were enough doctors to cover A&E, anyway. They hadn't had many patients come in, and the registrar didn't even have to do his own clerking of the uncomplicated cases, elderly falls and urinary tract infections.

You keep the children at a distance from you. You only use your travel mug for coffee and tea, and touch nothing without gloved hands.

You still feel like a fraud, though. You shouldn't. You have a fluctuating fever, muscle aches down to your elbows and knees, headache, no appetite, no energy, but you still feel like a fraud for being off sick. You message the team, and update them on your testing the next day, and realise that you're not really needed. When you're there, everyone else just works that much less. When you aren't, they work that much more, and the jobs still get done. Besides, it's an oddly quiet day on the ward. Looking at the list at home, there are fewer patients on the ward than you have ever seen.

You suppose you should use the time on mandatory sick leave in a useful way. You have an edit for your next children's book due, about brave brown girls solving another sinister mystery with medical-know-how. Your heroines do you what you cannot.

You have work to do for an editorial project on BAME representation in literature.

You have taxes.

You don't use the time usefully.

You sleep, and dream that you are back at the hospital, being useful.

Everyone is writing a diary, you realise. You are not the only scribe for your tribe. Nothing makes yours more meaningful, and you feel a surge of relief that you are writing this just for you. That someone else, someone fearless and eloquent, will do the job to publicise the shortcomings, the risks, the fears. All of this.

Your mother sends you that photo of your sister. Direct gaze to camera, hair cropped short, face shining and open. You had found it in a forgotten stack in your mum's kitchen, and took a shot on your rubbish little phone, and sent it around. It became the face of her WhatsApp funeral group, where everyone shared their thoughts and memories. It was the photo you sent to friends and colleagues when she died, with the tribute to her. On her birthday, you posted it with her most flattering chemo photo, from when she was bald and gorgeous, glamorous in a way she avoided in real life when she could be found hiding in owl-like glasses and oversized cardigans wrapped around her own knees. She had hated being dismissed for being pretty, you all are aware of the choices that beauty takes away.

There is no comment on the photo, and you don't know why your mother sent it, whether it was intended or a mistake. There is no anniversary, nothing like that. And nobody in the family group comments on it. It travels lightly around your family, seen and unremarked upon.

Hello, the photo says.

Hello, you reply. Unsure. You were always expecting her to tell you off about something. That feeling lingers, and you wonder how she'd feel about that. Relieved, maybe, that she still had that effect.

You had a good death, you tell her. You didn't think that at the time. All the miscommunication and misinformation. Your niece said they wouldn't have had a clue what was happening if you weren't a doctor. How the palliative team swept in and snorted when they heard your grade. You lost a lot of respect for the palliative speciality during that time, it felt like all their training had boiled down to writing up the same four medications and making the same sideways-cocked pity-face to whatever was asked and to whoever they were speaking.

A good death? she challenges.

We were all there, you said. Every day. We were there until the end. We all turned up for your god-squadding ceremonies and covered our hair, and we stood around your grave and prayed with our palms turned to the sky, and we went to your friends' house and ate trays of vegetable biryani.

Sounds like fun, she says. Wish I could've been there.

You were, you insist. You were there, and we were there, and when you left, we got to say goodbye. Nobody is getting to say goodbye anymore. They're dying alone.

And that's not a good death, she asks.

No, you say.

No, she says. It's a rebuke, a contradiction. So she had a great turn-out with two days' notice. It's not like she was able to appreciate it. She's telling you off again. Classic her.

You realise what she's saying. No death is a good death.

Don't look at the news, even though now you can. Don't watch the press briefing, even though now you've got the time.

15,000 deaths and counting.

84 deaths of workers in the health service. You're the new missionaries in the leper colonies. Except that leprosy, contrary to the fake news put about by biblical epic movies, is notoriously difficult to catch. And is now very treatable.

Lockdown is announced for another three weeks.

Three more weeks, people wail, they can't cope with their kids, with their lives within their four walls, and home is a prison, because any place is a prison if you can't leave.

Even heaven.

How's heaven working out for you? you ask your sister. You privately think it can't be that great if she's spending this much time in your head.

She's not going to answer that one.

That old lie. It is never good and sweet to die. Every death is a bad death.

24
Swab

It's day 28 of lockdown.

You're still sick. You're doing nothing. You're sleeping. You're sweating.

You're swabbed.

You do it yourself, in your car, in the drive-through testing area. You're only given one swab for both your throat and nose. It used to be two swabs, but the rules have changed in the two days you've been sick. You can't bring yourself to do the nose first, and then shove a snotty bogey-ridden bud down your throat. So you put it in your throat first, so deep that you cough, and the healthcare professionals who handed you the swab leap back, in their full PPE.

You go home and crawl back into the floor-bed, wiping handles you touched. You don't want to risk contaminating the kitchen, so you don't eat. You're not hungry, anyway.

That's all you've got. That's all you write.

It's day 29 of lockdown.

Still sick. Still doing nothing. Still sleeping. Sweating.

It's day 30 of lockdown.

Sick. Nothing. Sleep. Sweat.

That afternoon, you're out of bed.

Are you better? You must be feeling better. You drink coffee, which doesn't taste of anything. You go to the garden. Check your phone.

Result is back.

Covid detected.

You tell the kids.

No one can go out for fourteen days from when you got sick.

There are custard creams and fish fingers and apples and not much else.

The kids are delighted with the prospect of a fish finger and biscuit diet.

You thought they'd be terrified of you. But the worst thing that could happen has already happened. It's been happening for days, and everyone, apart from you, is fine.

You order a food delivery. You make a point of telling them to leave it on the front doorstep. Contact free.

It's day 31 of lockdown.

You're back in bed.

Sleeping. Sweating.

All your muscles ache. You're too tired to do anything. You can barely type this account. Every word marked down costs you something. Every step walked feels like an achievement.

You remember when you used to do stuff. How you used to chase away boredom and the risk of self-reflection with frenetic activity.

You're amazed how fast a day goes, when all you do is lie down.

The circle of the day isn't even punctuated by meals. You're still not eating.

The children are annoyed about keeping their distance. They want to hug you. They want to jump on the floor mattress that has become your sickbed. They want you to stop hogging the living room, as that's where the TV is, and watching it on their tablets isn't the same.

One week after you showed symptoms, you're theoretically clear to go back to work. The official line is just that you have to be symptom-free, other than a persisting cough, as that can take weeks to clear, even after you're proven Covid negative. You're expecting you'll be back at work soon. That the tiredness and the muscle ache and the fatigue and strange fog will all lift.

It is day 32 of lockdown and your chest is tight. That's new. When you try to breathe deeply, it is uncomfortable, almost painful, and you cough with instinctive irritation, causing a flurry of panic around the home.

MUMMYCOUGHED! MummyCOUGHED! Mummycoughed! Mummycoughed.

They repeat it to each other, and it echoes around your home in ever-decreasing circles.

It makes it easier to persuade them to keep their distance.

It is day 33 of lockdown, it is the end of April, although you are so tired you initially misdate this diary entry as somewhere in mid-June. Chest is still tight. Cough is more persistent. Fever flushes through you without warning. You're back in bed. You can't go to work like this. You email your apologies and feel guilty.

It is day 35 of lockdown. You can't wake up. You're drenched in sweat. You go back to sleep until lunchtime. You sit outside with the children. At a safe distance. You go back to bed. It's hard to breathe in, so you prone yourself like the bodies on ITU, lying flat on your stomach, to give your lung bases a chance to expand.

While you've been sick, the body count went past 20,000.

While you've been sick, Italy went past forty days of lockdown. *Quarantena*.

The original meaning of quarantine, forty days, feels big and biblical.

While you've been sick, Trump said out loud that ingesting or injecting bleach and sunlight should be explored by his researchers, while his medical advisor sat dumbly by, and didn't contradict him, like a kidnap victim afraid to blink twice for help.

While you've been sick, people have died in the US because they ingested or injected bleach.

While you've been sick, just three more weeks of lockdown became at least three more weeks of lockdown.

While you've been sick, the figures from Sweden, not locked down, rolled in with death after death after death.

While you've been sick, a sweet old man was promoted on BBC *Breakfast News* and his laps of his garden with his zimmer raised over 10 million pounds for the NHS, giving the government an excuse to deliver 10 million less that week.

While you've been sick, celebrities have been singing from their nicely decorated homes for charity and you've never really appreciated before quite how irrelevant they are, and why do we care about these people, why?

While you've been sick, you've avoided friends and family because you don't want to worry them and you can't deal with the concerns and the catastrophes and the Me-Me-Now-Ask-About-Me when you didn't ask them to ask about you in the first place.

While you've been sick, they said that each dead NHS worker is worth £60,000 to their family. That's what a family can claim for a relative who dies on the NHS frontline. So it turns out that you can put a price on sacrifice and it's pretty insulting.

This is the longest you've gone without writing.

This is the longest you've gone without working; even when you had the emergency C-section for your second twin you were back teaching at masters level within the week.

This is the longest you've gone without hugging the children, but your friends and family still judge you for sharing the same space, for walking into the kitchen to make your tea in your travel flask, for using the only toilet to pee.

This is the longest you've gone without washing your hair, you don't have the energy, even though it's grubby and itchy. You don't want to swill the virus from your contaminated surfaces around the bathroom.

You don't join the family Zoom, but you call your mother and complain about having Covid instead, and all the circumstances which conspired for you to catch it, and the children judge your language. You try and join your girlfriends' weekly WhatsApp with a glass of wine, and it tastes rank, everything tastes like crap or doesn't taste of anything at all.

People complain about stupid things like living without hairdressers, about hair going grey, and when you don't join the conversation they try and draw you in, with a What do you do about it? and you have to admit that you've cut your own hair for the last ten years, by tying it up into bunches and then cutting them off, that you don't colour your hair, that the only grey you've had is the same one you've had since childhood, in the same position where all your children have their single silver hair, and your sister's children too.

And they look at you disbelievingly and maybe they're thinking, Bitch.

You're not a kind person when you're sick.

You weren't that attractive when you were younger, but now you're in an unnaturally elongated prime. Your world is becoming smaller, closing and folding about you, and you criticise the edges of it, caustically. You curl up into yourself, and you care for so little beyond the frayed borders of self that it is frightening.

The day rockets past so fast when you sleep. You don't remember ever doing anything else. Being awake is the inconvenient bit, but it doesn't last long.

You realise that being ill has made you like everyone else in lockdown.

It is day 36. You wake up later and later each day, force yourself through the Covid fog to check the children have eaten something for breakfast, instruct them to drag a comb through their hair and then collapse on the sofa while they go through their school's allotted tasks for the morning. You take an hour to make and drink a cup of tea. You yell at them about large and small things, like kindness to each other, while you are struggling to summon that for yourself.

You listen to the radio and hear someone defending Trump about the bleach, as though it wasn't his fault, as his petrified bunny-in-the-headlights medical advisor hadn't contradicted him mid press conference.

You hear that NHS services might start running again, in some places. Outpatient clinics, perhaps. It's not clear.

You watch stupid stuff online. Light comedy on TV with the family. Nobody has the energy for a film. No one has the focus.

You wonder if you will miss this. Sitting at home with them. Watching TV. Cut off from the rest of the world. It's only been a week and you are fearful about rejoining the real world, you do not know if you'll be able to do your job, if you'll remember anything at all when the virus uncoils from your lung architecture.

Your children's father sees your tightness of breath and offers his inhaler.

That won't work, you explain. The inhaler is a beta2-agonist, it acts on the beta2 receptors in the smooth muscles of the lungs, helping them open. But the virus is actually sitting on the angiotensin II receptors bilaterally in the lung bases. You're surprised you remember anything medical at all.

You see a note that there will be new F1 doctors, rushed through graduation, with no elective or holiday, on the wards that day. You're still the F1 doctor, you haven't been moved ahead with your extra service star on your badge. Maybe they won't need you. It feels hard to quantify what you have achieved during a year as a doctor.

You're getting better. You ate half a crumpet. Half a bowl of ice cream. You're going to get up one day, and wash your hair and dress. You're going to pick up your bag and kiss your children goodbye and walk to work.

An article you wrote for a glossy magazine comes out, and readers post it online. It's you in scrubs, a selfie you had taken in the bathroom while you were waiting for a mandated medical teaching session. You can't remember why you took it. The lighting is terrible. Perhaps you'd wanted to show something to your mum. Your fringe trim. The main photo across the page fold is of a corridor, a stock shot of some kind of hospital. It looks like there are bars on some of the doors. Maybe a secure psych unit.

You had written that you wanted more people to join the NHS. It seems full of silly cup-half-full optimism, although you had been oddly prescient, writing months ago about suiting up to care for virus victims. You hadn't been writing about Covid, but the other common winter viruses, but everyone will assume you are.

Your piece is one of many, floating on the internet or stamped on shiny paper. The Covid-recovering GP without PPE talks for you, too. The psychogeographer writes beautifully about the multi-narrative structure of the pandemic, authored by the many. So many stories slipping through our fingers. Rippling past us like a hand in cool water. Searching for that elusive strand of truth.

Did you leave him? your sister asks. I thought you'd have left him by now.

She'd told you to do that, when she was dying. Her sort-of dying wish. Undiluted by diplomacy, edged with contention, like she was. Perhaps she was being control-ling, or kind, or both. Perhaps she liked the drama of it.

You tell her, There was never a good time.

You don't use a sister's funeral to announce a separation, it's about as tacky and me-me-me as using a friend's wedding to announce your baby.

Ross and Rachel did that, she points out.

You don't remember the old plot lines; other people are more up to date, watching it on Netflix with all the millennials. Hopeful and ironic. The show now seems so, so white. And all the women of colour were forced to date Ross.

So not at the funeral, and not after the funeral. Because then there was the sadness, and then there was her birthday, and then it was lockdown, day zero to now, almost forty days later. You couldn't leave each other, and so you just carried on, in the same house, simply absent from each other.

You and him. Her and you.

There was never a good time, you repeat.

Maybe that means there's never a bad time, either, she says. You're not sure if that neat illogic is hers or yours. It sounds like something that you would say.

I've been thinking about death, you say. Well duh. Seems a bit beside the point, saying that out loud. Like FaceTiming someone you see every day in real life. Death is all around. It's everywhere, and the air is constantly crackling with the expired electricity of it. The sound of breaking hearts is deafening. The new figures today are 40,000.

Some 20 per cent of all the worldwide deaths from Covid have happened in the UK. Is that right? That can't be right.

More civilians dead than the ones killed in the Blitz.

The Queen's mother looking the East End in the face, because she'd been bombed, too.

Who's looking you in the face?

Work are checking in with you, urging you to seek help if it gets worse. They're worried about you. You're in the demographic that dies. You wonder if they're worried you'll sue. Your hospital, like all hospitals, didn't have adequate PPE. Your ward wasn't meant to have had Covid-positive patients. Although of course you did.

You had Covid-positive healthcare workers, too.

You were one of them.

It was days until you realised you were actually sick, and it wasn't just the paranoia in your head making you feel so fearful.

The kids are chatting among themselves, casually gaming, and they point out that everyone dies. The alternative would be horrible. Like a zombie apocalypse, they say, pulling slack-jaw faces, holding their arms straight out in front of themselves in a grabby-zombie style and staggering with an undead limp.

Months ago, at the end of the summer, you were walking to work, and you saw that fox basking in the field not so far from the roadside.

The next day it was still there.

The day after you realised it wasn't sleeping, but dead.

And that was the week she told you she was dying.

And you watched the corpse of the fox every day, as it became something unrecognisable, clothed by the weeds over sinew and bone.

You can barely see him now; he's been so entangled and buried by the living greenery around him, feeding on his decay.

You see him most clearly in your thoughts.

The thought fox. Like the poem by Hughes.

He carries a burden in death he never did in life. We all do. We give away that thing we most need.

This is a story without a centre. And it has no natural end. Not even death can end it. This is our story.

Some tosser will tell the story from the virus's point of view, she says. With the virus as the hero.

And with death as the antagonist, you agree.

A part of you, seeking out the fox every morning, is worried that one day it will no longer be there.

For you, it's tied up into the tapestry of your sister's final illness and death, that summer's end as it lay plumply in the sunshine of the field, already dead or dying.

A part of you is worried that when the fox goes, she will go too.

How much of this is true? she asks. We want to know.

Why?

We want to know if it matters. And you know what you're like. Always bigging yourself up.

You're flattered she thought you bigged yourself up. You always thought you were small. You know you are small.

It always matters, you say. Everything matters.

You'd planned a whole monologue about this, before you got sick, but that was then, and you can no longer remember. Covid brain. It was probably a good speech, though. She'd have liked it. She liked the poem you wrote for her.

Now, you're falling asleep over the keyboard, and when you wake, she's not there, and you're speaking to the air. Your own words echoing back to you.

Everything matters. And everything is true.

★★★

You're better. Walking to work in the sunshine, along the dual carriageway, beside the stripped fields. Making a wide berth for the increasing numbers of joggers and the cyclists. You were sick for a couple of weeks. You didn't need to go back just yet, but you do, a few days early.

Your colleagues and your patients are keeping you busy. It's the bank holiday for VE Day, but everyone is working in the hospital. There are rumours about the end of lockdown, and people in a village are doing the conga, people are meeting up in parks, in the sunshine. Sharing benches and gin and tonics and bottles of champagne.

There's no vaccination as yet. No antibody test as yet, although it's on its way. The worst death rate in Europe. Forty days of lockdown. Forty thousand deaths and counting. They say this will double by the end of May.

In a few days, the prime minister will appear on the small screen waving his fists about like a squalling tyrant of an unjust regime. He will spout platitudes and confusing changes, telling people to try to go back to work on a few hours' notice, to not take public transport, as though that is any sort of option. Cannon fodder, the walking-working classes. No trying without dying.

The trains are packed on Monday, and there is nothing to do but wait. There will be another spike. The countdown is starting.

A patient is dying quietly, peacefully, on the ward. She isn't fit to go to the hospice. She wouldn't know where she was if she did. She is Covid positive.

Another patient is fighting against the night, he will not go quietly. He is young. He has cancer. He's dying, too.

You've turned away, when you approach the place where the fox lay. You don't want to see it anymore. You just want to let it go. To let go.

It's hard enough to lose life, to lose love, without watching it decay, day by day.

You look towards the hospital instead, emerging beyond the hill like a ship rising over the horizon.

This is what you wanted to do.

This is an extraordinary time.

This moment, these moments, will be made irrelevant by what is to come. The story isn't over yet, it is still unfolding, even as you write these final words.

She would never have believed this story as you have told it. You know that. But everything is true.

Epilogue – Poem for Kiron

The *Qul* for my sister, resting in the ground
Forever. Now. The gathering. The prayers
My sister says her name. She gives it to me
Something I have lost and she has found

She tells me the truth, it's too late to be sad
The bomb has fallen, the cloud has risen
But we're still grovelling in the dirt, scratching
Buried like bone, planted with stone

She tells me what she believes is true
Life goes on, she says, it must
The flesh has melted into the earth
But we're still rocking, banging on the floor

We washed her body, with gloved hands
If she had died a martyr
She would already be clean
But she was a woman, like me

Wrapped in white. A rock for a pillow
Head pointed west. Laid to rest
She was a believer, and we have no choice
You must be good for the dead

We believe. We have a choice
I choose the living. I, I, I choose life
And as we split open and weep
The walls tumble down like sheets

And blood bursts from torn skin
Like poppies on broken ground
My bond. My body. My blood
We go on. We must

The room is crumpled around us
The concrete beneath is cracked
We stand, exposed and weak
Newborn, washed by grief

Her body. Her blood. Buried. Beloved.
Faithful at the last. Gift-wrapped for God
She loved you, we tell them. We shine
With fragile hope, She loves you still

She leads us from the dark
She steps in a circle of light
We leave this pious place in line
With those who, like us, survived

Author's Note

Any piece such as this, written in the now, poured from real experiences during each of those first forty days of lockdown, has to be presented as a kind of autofiction as much as memoir to protect the confidentiality and privacy of patients and colleagues, as is my duty and their right.

And so I have changed names and details and perhaps have blasphemed by imagining and re-imagining what could not be told outright. The water re-forms and takes the shape of the vessel in which it is presented.

I think this isn't a story, so much as a romance. The account of relationships, between those who care and are cared for, between those who love, does not dare to veer from the truth. And as Hawthorne said, describing the writer's responsibility, would sin unpardonably if it did.

Acknowledgements

Grief is the long shadow cast by love. I started this book for my sister, Kiron. I finished it for all of us, for everyone who has lost someone they love.

With heartfelt thanks to those NHS colleagues, patients, friends and family who have taken this journey with me. And to Alexandra Pringle and Allegra Le Fanu at Bloomsbury, and Catherine Pellegrino at Marjacq, for encouraging me to share our stories.

A Note on the Type

The text of this book is set in Bembo, which was first used in 1495 by the Venetian printer Aldus Manutius for Cardinal Bembo's De Aetna. The original types were cut for Manutius by Francesco Griffo. Bembo was one of the types used by Claude Garamond (1480–1561) as a model for his Romain de l'Université, and so it was a forerunner of what became the standard European type for the following two centuries. Its modern form follows the original types and was designed for Monotype in 1929.